Service Standards for the NHS Care of Older People

A HEALTH SERVICES ACCREDITATION PUBLICATION
SPONSORED BY THE CENTRE FOR POLICY ON AGEING
FEBRUARY 1999

D1620890

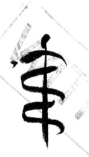

HEALTH SERVICES
ACCREDITATION

**Service Standards for
the NHS Care of Older People**

Citation details:
Health Services Accreditation (1999)
Service Standards for the NHS Care of Older People

ISBN 1 901097 45 5

Typeset by Jane Balshaw

Layout and design by Ivan Lee

Printed by The Weald Press Ltd

Health Services Accreditation
Rutherford Park
Marley Lane
Battle
East Sussex TN33 0EZ

Tel: (01424) 772277
Fax: (01424) 774477
eMail: info@nhs-accreditation.co.uk
Web: http://www.nhs-accreditation.co.uk

Centre for Policy on Ageing
25 -31 Ironmonger Row
London EC1V 3QP

Tel: 0171 253 1787
Fax: 0171 490 4206
eMail: cpa@cpa.org.uk

The Centre for Policy on Ageing, established in 1947 by the Nuffield
Foundation, is an independent organisation which seeks to promote
the interests of older people through research, information and the
spread of good practice in health and social welfare services. In
addition to its policy and research work, the Centre has an
internationally renowned library collection on older age issues, an
information service that produces AgeInfo CD-ROM, and an active
publishing programme.

Contents

Page

Improving health care through Health Services Accreditation

WELCOME TO HEALTH SERVICES ACCREDITATION

The report you are about to read is one of a growing range of titles focusing on areas of patient care across the entire health service. It has been prepared by a working group drawing on input from service provider professionals, commissioners, general practitioners, service managers and, most importantly, lay representation.

WHAT SERVICE STANDARDS REPORTS CONTAIN

A Health Services Accreditation (HSA) service standards report presents, in one volume, a compendium of essential service standards focused on a specific area of care. It is the prototype of the National Service Frameworks described in the quality Green Papers (1998). Having cast their net across published research, benchmarked practice, consensus opinion, tradition and innovation, our working groups offer their reports as practical guides to the key issues currently impacting on quality of service in each area considered.

Their reports refer to statutory and Patient's Charter rights and standards and include recommendations and obligatory requirements from Royal Colleges and the national bodies representing other health care professionals and patients. Among other key topics each report addresses essential and appropriate clinical audit; risk management; integrated care pathway development; team working; the introduction of evidence based practice, and organisational issues (including policy, procedures, training and education).

In other words, this report aims to provide an authoritative but imaginative survey and analysis of its service area. It sets out an overall, prioritised national framework for a quality service whilst not forgetting essential detail. In the view of the working group producing it, a view reached after profound study and very wide consultation, it contains what you want to know, what you ought to be doing and what you need to be thinking about. Look on it as a friendly guide through the service quality maze and the basis for your programme towards clinical governance in geriatric medicine.

BEFORE YOU BEGIN. . .

Before you begin to read and use this report there is one key point HSA would like to leave with you. This report is not designed to stand alone. It is an integral part of a process designed to help you get its contents off the bookshelf and into practice.

The HSA programme offers you a user-friendly method for tackling the prime issues raised in this report. Within a simply structured process, it takes you step by step from your own assessment of your current service to the identification of any service improvement needs. It enables you to clearly determine just what needs to be done and how.

And while this is under way, evidence is generated which authenticates and validates the quality of your service and provides the information necessary to meet your audit, monitoring and accreditation responsibilities.

SO WHAT IS HSA?

The Health Services Accreditation approach to aiding and assuring quality in health care is based upon five principles:

First of these is its approach to providing an integrated, holistic programme for prioritising, co-ordinating and implementing quality in healthcare.

Second, HSA addresses each service area from the perspective of the patient's experience of it. Care services increasingly rarely fit within single organisational boundaries and a meaningful approach to quality through standards must do the same.

Third, the HSA programme is building a comprehensive portfolio of service standards to address principal service areas across primary, secondary and community care, incorporating clinical as well as organisational issues and those concerns which research shows colour the patient's personal experience.

Fourth, the HSA programme is national in scope and applicability. It promotes a genuinely national health service through standards requiring equity of provision and access at geographical and individual levels.

Fifth, HSA is committed to fair, achievable and objective measures of structure, process and performance and a transparent and robust method for validating achievement and placing quality information in the public domain.

THE HSA PROGRAMME

How does HSA put these principles into practice? As we have shown above, our service standards reports are fundamental to the process.

Drawn from these reports are their companion accreditation instruments. In these all the most salient features of their corresponding reports are defined in statements which characterise aspects of a quality service (see annex A).

These statements are expressed as either MINIMUM or BEST PRACTICE. Minimum represents what is deemed essential for a safe and effective service. Best practice takes us into areas of innovation and excellence.

Backing up each of these defined characteristic statements are specific elements or features of service provision or measurement. These are expressed as standards (supported by items of evidence required) which together, if achieved, justify the application of the statement to your service (see annex B).

Accreditation instruments therefore not only provide a working manual for providers to map service improvement needs but offer an agenda for priority action which also spells out what that action should be. They serve as the explicit and objective instrument for the validation of your achievement.

3

A STRAIGHTFORWARD AND OPEN PROCESS

Services participating in the HSA programme begin with internal self-assessment against the accreditation instrument, to determine where they stand and what needs to be done. As they work through this development programme they are at the same time producing the evidence required to confirm their achievement. In due course they invite HSA to test, evaluate and confirm this evidence. This done, HSA issues a statement setting out which standards are found to apply. Details of this simple process are found in other HSA publications, available on request from the HSA office.

HOW YOU CAN SHARE IN THE BENEFITS OF HSA

In this straightforward but carefully crafted package, service standards report, accreditation instrument and process to verify the achievement of standards combine to offer a dynamic approach to defining, implementing and confirming care service quality.

* Providers are effectively enabled to translate standards into practice in a co-ordinated continuous quality improvement programme which forms a sound basis for clinical governance

* Commissioners of care find it a key tool to help focus commissioning intentions and ensure the availability of vital and relevant quality information

* The interested public gain access to factual and meaningful information on what really matters in their health service, and how well it is being provided

If, having read this report, you would like to learn more of how the HSA programme can aid you achieve these goals, please contact:

Mrs Jan Dowlen
Director

If you wish to assist HSA in its own continuous quality improvement programme, we welcome your views and comments on the contents of this document. Please write to:

Tony Jenkins
Director of Standards Development

Your views and comments on HSA accreditation materials and the HSA assured accreditation process will be welcome contributions to our own efforts towards quality improvement. Please send them to:

Martin Savage
Director of Accreditation

Health Services Accreditation
Rutherford Park
Marley Lane
Battle
East Sussex TN33 0EZ
Tel: (01424) 772277   Fax: (01424) 774477   eMail: info@nhs-accreditation.co.uk

Foreword

This is the second report on Service Standards for the NHS Care of Older People produced by Health Services Accreditation. The first, published in 1994, was one of the earliest in the HSA series of service standards reports addressing important areas of patient care. Work on the second edition began in 1996, with a reconvened working group of new and former members, chaired by Dr Gillian Dalley, Director of the Centre for Policy on Ageing. Dr Dalley was formerly Quality Manager of the South East Thames Regional Health Authority, and took a prominent role there in the development of service standards and accreditation before taking up her present post. Her understanding of standard setting, and her concern with all aspects of policy affecting older people, have been invaluable in steering the group towards agreement on key standards for the quality of care received by this section of the population. Both the HSA report Focus on Patients, and other work involving groups of older people, also informed the working group's response to the areas covered in this volume. The work of researching, drafting and editing the standards for the care of older people report has been undertaken with enthusiastic and consistent commitment by Sarah Hadley of HSA who also facilitated the preparation of Focus on Patients.

Agreeing the parameters for a report such as this is difficult. A number of comments on the draft report during consultation noted the omission of standards for care in nursing and residential homes. Work addressing these areas is currently being undertaken for the Department of Health by the Centre for Policy on Ageing, and should be available during 1999.

Effective joint working and the prompt delivery of services is often crucial to an older person's experience of care. The difficulties of multi-agency provision, most particularly by health and social services, is recognised in the Government's recent discussion document Partnership in Action. Implementation of proposals for pooled budgets, lead commissioners and integrated provision should enable greater flexibility in providing effective health and social care and lead to the achievement of the standards in this report. The way forward outlined in the White Paper The New NHS, and in particular the setting up of primary care groups (PCGs), will add momentum to the drive to improve community based services. The Green Paper, A First Class Service, and its companions for Wales and Scotland, signal an increasing emphasis on the quality of NHS services. This report is intended as a contribution to the achievement of that goal.

Finally we should again like to thank the members of the working group, our colleague Martin Savage, the HSA staff and the many individuals and organisations who responded in great detail to the report in draft, for their contributions and support. Their thoughtful and constructive comments made an important contribution to the final document.

A C Jenkins
Director of Standards Development
Health Services Accreditation

Executive summary

Section 1   Outlines the context for delivery of services to older people; indicates the scope of the report and the principles that should govern the provision of care.

Section 2   Examines health and social care available in the community including the organisation and delivery of services, access, standards for home visits, assessment and care planning. The report focuses on the need for multi-professional integrated joint service team work. Standards for risk management, health and safety and health promotion are also included.

Section 3   Introduces standards for the care of the older person when presenting at A&E, on admission, and as an inpatient. Particular issues such as pain management, nutrition, ward facilities and staffing are among those examined. The section also sets standards for outpatient services, day hospital and rehabilitation services. The importance of multi-disciplinary cross-boundary team work is stressed throughout.

Section 4   Concentrates on the need for applied communication policies which link patients, carers, primary and secondary care and social care agencies. Topics addressed include referral practice, record keeping, and discharge (transfer of care) communication. The role of carers is emphasised and standards are recommended for a Hospital at Home scheme.

Section 5   Deals with consent, confidentiality, privacy and dignity and complaints procedures. The impact of these issues on the patient's view of the NHS is emphasised. Particular needs of members of ethnic groups are examined. Guidance for action on suspected elder abuse, both domestic and institutional, is given. Key features of care of the terminally ill are covered.

Section 6   Looks at strategies for preventing avoidable falls by older people both within the community and in the acute care environment.

Section 7   This section looks at the incidence and pathology of dementia. It examines the management of dementia in the community and in the acute sector. Strategies are proposed to increase true awareness of the condition and to manage its treatment and/or the care of patients with a dementia syndrome.

Section 8   The management of patients with stroke serves as a valid proxy for the care of the older person, raising questions of the application of evidence based practice, the necessity for clear quality standards applying to inpatient care, discharge and follow-up/rehabilitation and the clinical audit of services delivered. Each aspect is considered and standards which define safe and effective care are specified.

Section 9   Section 9 introduces and explains the importance of routine, systematic clinical multi-professional audit of the delivery of care to older persons. It sets out standards for the organisation and management of audit programmes and key topics which should feature in the audit of care provided in the acute and community sectors.

1 Introduction

At the time of our going to press the Health Advisory Service 2000 published their report Not Because They Are Old: an independent enquiry into the care of older people on acute wards in general hospitals (November 1998). Readers will find our standards report addresses both the concerns identified and the recommendations made in the HAS document. HAS 2000 calls for 'a National Service Framework for Older People, made up of key indicators of quality care and service provision. . . to ensure the profile and priority given to older people is raised and maintained.' The clear need for such a document extending through acute services and into the community has inspired HSA's work in this field throughout, and we are delighted therefore to be able to make our national service framework for older people available to colleagues in the NHS and other care providers. Its publication could not be more timely in the context of HAS 2000's work and the introduction of Clinical Governance. We hope that colleagues will find it a helpful, useful and readable aid towards maintaining and improving the quality of care delivered to older people.

1.1 CONTEXT FOR PROVISION

This report addresses standards of health services for older people and related issues of social care relevant to an increasing proportion of the population. One in six of the population is now a pensioner. More significantly for the health service, the number of people aged over 85 has doubled since 1981. The challenge of the increased longevity achieved during this century is highlighted in a recent Audit Commission report, The Coming of Age[1]. Longevity, states the report, must be accompanied by adequate finances, fitness and good health, so that the quality of life is maintained for both older people and their families. Maintaining good health requires active care, preventing ill-health wherever possible, providing active rehabilitation after illness and getting the right support where health is failing.

The recent green paper issued by the Government, A First Class Service, which sets out a central role for the introduction of quality standards and monitoring, provides the national context for the delivery of a high standard service[2].

The growth in the proportion of older people in the population is taking place against a background of major political changes during the 1990s to both the funding and provision of care for older people. The transfer of responsibility for funding of people in residential and nursing homes from the Department of Social Security (DSS) to local authorities, together with cut-backs in local authority expenditure, led to radical changes in the provision of long term care for older people, with the private and voluntary sectors playing a major role in the provision of nursing and residential care as well as home care services. Many of these agencies, together with the NHS, are seeking to strengthen links with other service providers. However the scope of this report is primarily intended for those providing a service to older people within the NHS, albeit in association with other agencies, particularly social services.

In line with the increased emphasis on community based health care, social service departments are being encouraged to develop a more therapeutic approach to the care of older people and to challenge commonly held assumptions about the inevitability of disability and dependence[3]. Likewise community based NHS services seek to support older people in their wish to retain their independence.

Local eligibility criteria for continuing care and in some cases care in the community are jointly agreed with social services[4]. The new powers of local authorities to arrange nursing and residential home placements has introduced means testing for many. Others requiring continuing care may or may not meet the criteria for NHS funded continuing care. The result has been not only to restrict the provision of NHS provided care but to render it inequitable across the country, creating a situation of complexity and confusion for patients and the public.

Health and local authorities need to ensure that the criteria for assessments for NHS continuing care and for means tested residential care are clearly understood by professionals and the public, who should also be informed of the appeals procedure.

These changes have had a direct impact on both health and social care in terms of access, cost and quality for older people and their carers and for those trying to provide a comprehensive service to meet their needs. The devolution of provision, and decisions on the commissioning of services, carries the risk of increasing deprivation in some areas as does the absence of a broad perspective for the planning of future services and adherence to the principle of equity of access in health care.

1.2   SCOPE OF THE REPORT

Whilst this report focuses on standards of health care for older people, there are, inevitably, other areas that relate closely to health issues. Since joint working between the NHS and social services is so important, a number of social issues are referred to in this report.

The people who are the central focus of this report may be described predominantly, although not exclusively, as those over the age of 75 and others aged over 65 who have multiple and complex needs.

Geriatric medicine evolved in the 1950s and 1960s, from the realisation that many elderly people in institutional care had not received appropriate investigation or rehabilitation, to its present position as the central plank of a multi-disciplinary approach to the diagnosis and treatment of acute and chronic diseases that affect older people. This report concentrates on standards for this service, encompassing the care of older people in the full range of health care settings where they access services.

The standards for acute/secondary care set out in this document focus on the special needs of older people. General standards defining the quality issues arising in acute/secondary care are found in HSA's reports on Standards for Emergency Surgical Services, Accident and Emergency Services, and Emergency Medical Admissions. Therefore services for older people seeking to ensure overall quality should aim to achieve at least the minimum standards in the relevant service area (surgery, medicine or A&E) together with the standards in this volume.

An important standard for services for older people is the ability of patients to access other specialties in acute and community services where these are necessary. The needs of older people receiving treatment in other parts of the health service are referred to in various HSA reports. Thus Standards for A&E Services[5], Service Standards for Discharge Care[6] and others contain particular standards for the care of older people. Where relevant these will be referred to and expanded as appropriate.

A separate report on standards for adult mental health services is being prepared by Health Services Accreditation (HSA) and will deal with standards for the elderly mentally ill in detail. This present report, however, considers dementia and access to elderly mentally ill (EMI) services.

Providing support to carers may be crucial to enabling the older person to remain at home. Other issues such as housing and financial problems, although their resolution will usually involve other organisations, can impact on the health and ability of older people to remain independent. Health professionals should be aware of the circumstances of the older person and how these might influence their physical and psychological well-being.

1.3   PRINCIPLES UNDERLYING SERVICES TO OLDER PEOPLE

Health service professionals have a responsibility to provide the same quality of treatment and care to older people as they would to any other patient group, albeit there are pressures, particularly the limited resources available, which may militate against the provision of a full range of care. Trust policies refusing access to certain services on the grounds of age alone have on occasion received well publicised and critical attention in the media. The working group therefore recommends that Trust policies should clearly state that no services will be refused to patients solely on the grounds of age. Particular importance is attached to the following principles that should underlie service provision in order to ensure equitable provision of care for older people:

a. Older people are entitled to the full range of health care free at the point of delivery, according to their clinical need, in common with users of the NHS
b. Older people have an equal right to investigation and management as all other age groups
c. Older people should be able to access health provision even where this is not locally based (for instance specialist care)
d. The range of health and social care provided should be experienced by the patient as seamless, that is as a service fully integrated between provider agencies
e. Older people should be enabled to make informed choices about their treatment and the location of their care
f. Older people should be supported in their desire to lead as full and independent a life as possible
g. The burden of care on families and other care givers should not exceed that which is comfortably tolerable to them given their circumstances
h. Iatrogenic insult should be avoided in the application of all health measures

2 Services in the community

2.1 THE NHS AND THE COMMUNITY CARE ACT (1990) AND THE PROVISION OF COMMUNITY BASED SERVICES

The provision of services in the community by the NHS and by local authorities is an essential part of the government's strategy for providing community care to meet health and social care needs. Social services departments have a lead role under the NHS and Community Care Act 1990 in the planning and purchasing of social care to meet the needs of the local population and of individuals. Hence social services must be involved in the assessment of individual needs for personal social services.

2.1.1 From April 1996 health authorities have been required to develop local policies and eligibility criteria for entitlement to NHS funded continuing care. Such criteria must be agreed with local authorities and other relevant agencies[7],[4] and include a procedure for the resolution of disputes.

2.1.2 These two aspects of government policy, designed to achieve a spectrum of health and social care, provide the framework for the provision of community based health and social care. Implementation of policy will require common assessment documentation shared between health and social services. It is important that health service staff should be aware of the available social care services and that social services staff should have an understanding of effective healthcare interventions and an individual's potential for rehabilitation.

2.1.3 Joint assessment of care planning is covered by agreements between health authorities, NHS Trusts and local authorities, including social services and housing. These agreements centre on:

    a. Hospital discharge arrangements: these should include guidance for referral to other agencies; response times for referral; a requirement to identify a key worker responsible for implementation of the care plan

    b. Agreed criteria for NHS continuing care: this involves service definitions for health and social care

    c. Local eligibility for care in the community: as with (b) above this requires service definitions for health and social care and eligibility for accessing services

2.1.4 The aim of services in the community is to establish a comprehensive range of services that will give support to older people when it is needed, in order to enable them to remain at home if that is their wish. The 1990 NHS and Community Care Act introduced changes in the organisation of community care services. Local authority social service departments were given lead responsibility for community care, working with health and housing departments to ensure the provision of integrated services. The actual provision of social care however, could come from the independent sector, purchased by local authorities.

2.1.5 Community based health care is primarily provided by general practitioners, community health services, district nurses, health visitors, therapists and specialist nursing services. Secondary care providers also provide community based care such as psychiatry of old age, rehabilitation services and in some instances, rural community hospitals. Social services and independent agencies also have a role. The introduction of primary care groups (PCGs) proposed in the White Paper[8], which it is proposed shall include representatives from the health authority, social services and nursing, is a recognition of the importance of integrated provision.

2.1.6   The spectrum of care should include a focus on well being, proactive care and rehabilitation. It can range from a short period of support and rehabilitation following discharge from hospital, treatment and support to people who have chronic conditions, through to palliative care to enable the dying patient to remain at home if he/she so wishes.

2.1.7   Community health services should also be provided to patients in residential homes. In some areas primary health care teams (PHCTs) have started to offer health promotion advice to staff in residential homes on issues such as communication difficulties, mobility, eating difficulties, continence and hygiene. Early intervention may result in a better managed workload for the team, which may have clinical responsibility for a number of patients in residential homes.

2.2   **REFERRAL TO COMMUNITY HEALTH SERVICES**

General practitioners are not only responsible for the provision of primary care services to the patient but also have access to hospital and community health services not provided by the PHCT. It is therefore essential that older people should be encouraged to register with a general practitioner.

2.2.1   General practitioners provide the most likely referral path to Community Trust services. The general practice should be aware of the key managerial contacts for these services and should know how to access them. Other referral routes to community services are through discharge from hospital; from one of the services listed in Box 1 below, or, in some cases, self referral by the patient[9]. The general practitioner must be informed of referrals received by other routes including cross referrals from outpatient clinics, and receive a written report of the assessments made of the patient within four working days. General practitioners may also be a key source of referral for local authority assessment and services. It is therefore essential that general practitioners and PHCT staff are aware of the procedures for such referral.

2.2.2   In all cases the reason for the referral should be understood by the patient and/or carer and the patient's consent obtained on the basis of an understanding of the available options. If the patient is unable to consent the health professional has a responsibility to act in the patient's best interest[10].

2.2.3   The referral letter/information must include the reason for referral, a brief medical history, the medication being taken, information on access to the home (if a home visit is needed); other relevant information such as sensory or cognitive impairment; reference to the need for an interpreter for visits to those without knowledge of English. Use of a standard referral form covering these aspects is recommended.

2.3   **SERVICES AVAILABLE IN THE COMMUNITY**

2.3.1   The underlying policy objective of the community care reforms has been to improve domiciliary care services so as to enable more people to be cared for at home, if that is their wish[11] or in a nursing or residential home if that is where they live. If this objective is to be achieved then a range of health and social care support needs to be available on a multi-disciplinary basis, their provision achieved through an established mechanism for effective communication between professionals, the patient and carer. These services are summarised in Box 1 below.

2.3.2   Social care, which includes home care services, respite care, meals on wheels, assistance with shopping, and day centres, is available through social services. Provision of these services is subject to local authority eligibility criteria and the individual may be charged, possibly after means testing, for the service. Accessible points of access to these services should be identified to service providers and the public.

BOX 1

Services available in the community should include:

a. 24-hour nursing services, including twilight and night nursing services
b. Specialist nursing services
c. Occupational therapy
d. Physiotherapy
e. Chiropody
f. Speech and language therapy (communication and swallowing management)
g. Continence advisory services
h. Specialist orthotics service
i. Community mental health team (CMHT) for the elderly
j. Counselling
k. Audiology
l. Optical services
m. Dentistry
n. Dietetics
o. Palliative care
p. Access to equipment loans
q. Wheelchair services
r. Health visiting
s. Pharmacy

2.4   THE GENERAL PRACTITIONER

2.4.1   The general practitioner and his/her team have a central role in the provision of health care to older people and it is therefore important that primary care provision demonstrates an awareness of the needs of this group of patients. The surgery design needs to facilitate access by the elderly, frail and disabled. Details of local parking facilities and public transport included in the practice information leaflet will assist patients wishing to visit the doctor. Regular review of repeat and multiple prescriptions and arrangements with pharmacists for the home delivery of medicines should be undertaken. Therapeutic areas to be audited include general practitioner prescribing for the elderly and the rehabilitation of older people after falls[12].

2.4.2   The general practitioner should be aware of the availability of certain NHS services such as audiology, ophthalmic services, dentistry, chiropody, speech and language therapy and physiotherapy, and know how these services can be accessed. Participation in programmes for prevention of falls, stroke etc., demonstrate a commitment to promoting a healthy independent lifestyle for older people. A number of these tasks can be done by other members of the primary health care team. However the general practitioner's role is to identify aspects of the service to older people which can be improved.

2.5   DISTRICT NURSING SERVICES

2.5.1   District nurses form the backbone of nursing care in the community. Patients may be referred to district nurses from a variety of sources e.g. general practitioner or hospital. District nurse services are generally day-time only, although increasingly areas are providing a twilight and night-time service[13]. The Marie Curie service, for example, provides nursing care on a 24-hour basis to cancer patients, and must liaise closely with local district nursing services in order to provide an integrated nursing service for patients at home. Alternative arrangements for night nursing must be made where the district nursing service is not provided on a 24-hour basis.

2.5.2   The district nurse is responsible for the nursing component of the care delivered by his/her team, initially completing a holistic nursing assessment of the patient. Referrals to other services may derive from this initial assessment. The subsequent care plan will be drawn up in conjunction with the patient, carers and other relevant professionals.

2.5.3   Specialist nursing for diabetic care, Parkinson's disease, palliative care, stoma care, continence and mental health should be included in the provision made by community nursing services or otherwise available for access by the district nurse team in response to patient need.

2.5.4   Response times for referrals to the district nurse differ according to the contract with service commissioners but usually an urgent referral will be actioned within two hours (Patient's Charter requirement is within four hours, see Box 6), and non urgent referrals within 48 hours unless a specified day is requested.

2.5.5   The district nursing service should be able to demonstrate how the service is meeting the needs of the local population.

2.6   THERAPY SERVICES

2.6.1   Services need to have locally agreed standards for responding to urgent and non-urgent referrals.

2.6.2   Occupational therapists may be employed by health or social services which will reflect health and social provision. In addition to assessment, occupational therapists have a role in providing treatment to improve and/or maintain functional independence. They also have a role in preventing admissions by intervening before a crisis arises. Most occupational therapists in the community are employed by either social services or acute and community trusts. They have a role in assessment as well as organising adaptations in the home and providing equipment maximising the safe, independent activity of the patient. The work of the occupational therapist is an important component in helping the patient retain independence on return home from hospital.

2.6.3   Physiotherapy, speech and language therapy, and chiropody all provide a service which can be essential for enabling older people to remain in their own home. Access to these services may vary between areas but is generally through the general practitioner, district nurse or hospital consultant.

2.6.4   There is considerable variation between health authorities in the range of chiropody services available. Increasingly, access to NHS chiropody services is based solely on an assessment of clinical need and a large proportion of the 'at risk' groups are older people. The general practitioner needs to be aware of what chiropody services are available and be able to advise where routine procedures, such as nail cutting, can be obtained from a qualified chiropodist if they are not provided by chiropody departments.

2.6.5   The main areas of responsibility of physiotherapists, occupational therapists, speech and language therapists and chiropodists are outlined in Box 2.

2.6.6   It should be noted that these services should be available on a domiciliary basis for the housebound at general practitioner request, as well as from clinics. The level of demand in most cases probably exceeds supply. It is therefore important that advice on preventative measures is given in order to avoid future problems as far as possible.

2.6.7   Therapy services, wherever located or employed, should seek to ensure they are able to maintain their staffing at a level which will allow them to cover annual leave and sickness periods without necessarily relying upon locum services.

2.7   DENTISTRY

2.7.1   Community dental services provide treatment for those who are unable to obtain treatment from a general dental practitioner. This particularly applies to older patients who are physically and/or mentally frail who may need a domiciliary visit. The priority for these patients is therapeutic dentistry. Prevention of dental problems is also important and this may require the co-operation of the carer. Requirements for a preventative approach in dental treatment are outlined in Box 3.

2.7.2   Trusts must not allow staffing levels in dentistry to fall below the level required to provide domiciliary emergency cover to older physically and/or mentally frail patients.

2.8   DIETETICS

2.8.1   Nutrition is an important aspect of a multi-disciplinary approach to the needs of the older person. Essential features of the community dieticians role are listed in Box 4.

BOX 2

Principle responsibilities of occupational therapists:

a. To assess patients in their own homes in order to identify factors which may affect independence in daily living
b. To plan and undertake a treatment programme
c. To organise equipment and home adaptations if required
d. To facilitate and work with carers in order to enable people to continue living at home

Principle responsibilities of the community physiotherapist are:

e. To improve mobility after hospitalisation for fractures or joint replacement and to prevent falls[14]
f. Help to restore mobility and confidence after a fall
g. Stroke rehabilitation and other neurological conditions
h. Dealing with acute musculoskeletal problems
i. Advice to patients to prevent muscle wasting
j. Advice to carers and nurses on safe moving and handling

Principal responsibilities of speech and language therapists:

k. To assess and manage communication problems
l. Assist with problems of feeding and swallowing
m. To actively involve carers in meeting the patient's communication and swallowing needs

Essential functions of the chiropodist[13]:

n. Treatment of foot problems such as foot ulcers, rheumatoid feet, nail problems
o. To provide advice on preventative measures and footwear
p. To attend to 'at risk' groups such as those with diabetes, peripheral vascular disease
q. To provide corrective orthoses for functional problems

BOX 3

Preventative dentistry for older patients includes:

a. Plaque control by means of proper, twice daily tooth-brushing using a fluoridated toothpaste (with help from carers if necessary)
b. A healthy diet with a reduction in the number of intakes of non-milk extrinsic sugars
c. Marking of all dentures, preferably during their construction but otherwise on admission to a hospital, or nursing/residential home
d. Avoidance of low pH artificial saliva in patients with any natural teeth
e. Annual dental examination including screening of the oral tissues

BOX 4

> **Community dieticians should provide:**
>
> a. Direct or indirect provision of dietary management for specific medical conditions
> b. Training and update to other professionals to enable an assessment of the nutritional needs of the patient
> c. Assessment tools to monitor the nutritional status of the patient
> d. Ensure that members of the multi-disciplinary team are aware of referral procedures to the dietetic service
> e. Liaison with general practitioners and pharmacists on use of nutritional supplements, laxatives etc
> f. Liaison with social services to advise on nutrition in, for example, meals on wheels, day centres

2.8.2   Community dieticians also have an important role in training nurses, catering and support staff at nursing and residential homes.

2.9   **PHARMACY**

A crucial issue for patients at home is obtaining advice and medication from the pharmacist. A number of community pharmacists deliver drugs to patients' homes. The HSA report on community pharmacy recommends standards for community pharmacists[15]. Included are standards for a system to ensure provision of information to the patient and/or carer on the correct and safe administration of medicines.

2.9.1   Pharmaceutical services are also provided by acute and community trusts and must provide advice to patients on how to take their medication. Detailed standards on achieving compliance are included in Standards for NHS Pharmacy in Hospital and Community Health Services[16]. Measures that should be considered by pharmacists to help older people are given in Box 5.

BOX 5

> **To obtain compliance with prescribed medication pharmacists should:**
>
> a. Advise the doctor on methods to simplify drug regimens
> b. Involve carers in the management of medication and advise about the benefits and purposes of medication as well as possible side-effects
> c. Consider providing the patient with loaded dosettes (plastic containers divided into days)
> d. Advise on use of a medication chart or daily dose reminder for patients on a number of drugs
> e. Consider providing drugs in non child-proof containers for those with limited manual dexterity, and large print labels for the visually impaired
> f. Notify the general practitioner in writing if compliance problems are suspected

2.9.2   The hospital pharmacy should have a priority system in place to identify discharge prescriptions requiring specific communication with the primary health care team (PHCT), including the community pharmacist, on subjects such as patients on complex drug regimes or those needing monitoring.

2.10   THE HOME VISIT

2.10.1   An initial risk assessment and assessment of care needs associated with the management of the patient's care should be carried out by the health professional who first visits the patient.

2.10.2   The Patient's Charter includes the following requirements relating to home visits[17] by representatives/providers of NHS services.

BOX 6

> **Patient's charter requirements for domiciliary visits by nurses:**
>
> **a.** Patients and/or carers should be consulted about a convenient time to visit
> **b.** The visit should take place within a two hour time band of the appointment time
> **c.** If the appointment cannot be kept the patient should be informed and another appointment arranged
> **d.** The community nurse (or CPN if indicated) should visit an urgently referred patient within four hours (during the day)
> **e.** Patients on non-urgent referral must be visited within two working days
> **f.** Visits should take place on the day asked for by the patient providing there is more than 48 hours notice

Where appropriate these Patient's Charter standards should be applied in consultation with the carer as well as the patient.

2.10.3   All professionals on home visits must show their identification card or badge. An additional reassurance to the older person, particularly those with poor eyesight, is to state clearly the name and title of the professional when the visit is being arranged. An identification card with contact number should be left. The patient and carer should be told the purpose of the visit in advance and again during the visit.

2.10.4   Professional associations have specific requirements relating to domiciliary visits. Speech and language therapists will accept referrals from any source providing that the patient's consent has been obtained. The therapist will have notified the relevant member of the multidisciplinary team with details of the planned visit. The initial assessment should include whether home visits are the best location for further interventions. The main case notes should be kept at the working location and record the home visit. The results of the assessment and proposed therapy plan must be communicated to the multi-disciplinary team.

2.10.5   The sharing of information between professionals caring for an older person is essential. Nevertheless the patient's permission for this sharing should be sought in the first instance and he/she should be made aware when other professional advice is being sought. Before the visiting professional leaves following a home visit, the patient should be told what the next stage in their care is, or could be, and the likely timescale. Use of patient-held records may facilitate communications (see also 2.13). Records should include written notes on the next steps to be taken.

2.10.6   Each visit must include an explanation to the patient of the outcome. A written summary of visits should be made and copied to the care manager. This may also be left with the patient unless alternative action is advised in guidance to staff, e.g. if elder abuse is suspected. Protocols must be in place for dealing with urgent problems or changes in treatment that impact on the care plan.

2.10.7   A local procedure must be in place on what action should be taken in the event of any unexpected incident or emergency during a home visit. These should include contacting the police or emergency services if necessary. In particular the inability to get a reply on an arranged visit must be attended to at the time and reported to the line manager and/or key worker.

2.10.8   Domiciliary visits (DVs) by a consultant may take place jointly with the general practitioner who has requested advice on diagnosis and treatment. Pre-admission DVs may sometimes result in hospital admission being avoided[44]. A home visit may give the clinician clearer background knowledge for future management plans. The British Geriatrics Society (BGS) has suggested guidelines for the most effective use of domiciliary visits to patients, and the following proposals are based[18] on these.

BOX 7

Guidelines for domiciliary visits by consultants:

a. Use of referral form to access information supplied by the general practitioner, including details on access to the premises
b. Direct contact between consultant and general practitioner prior to visit
c. The patient's consent is required for other staff or students to be present
d. The consultant is required to communicate the outcome and recommendations following the visit, to the general practitioner
e. The patient and carers must be notified of the outcome of the visit either by the consultant or general practitioner

---

2.10.9   The time scales for making urgent and non-urgent domiciliary visits by consultants must be agreed between the Trust and purchaser, who may be the general practitioner. The patient's consent should be obtained if trainees, medical students and/or nursing staff wish to attend.

2.11   **ASSESSMENT FOR CARE IN THE COMMUNITY**

Health and local authorities have been asked to develop a framework for multi-disciplinary assessment in community and acute settings[19]. This can be seen as a first step towards the Government's intention of removing legislative barriers to enable integrated care provision.

2.11.1   The key to the proper targeting and delivery of care is a thorough assessment of the patient's needs. The DoH has outlined requirements to achieve Better Services for Vulnerable People in EL(97)62[20]. This includes indicators for good multi-disciplinary assessment, as follows:

a. A clearly identified purpose for the assessment
b. Effective screening/trigger mechanisms to ensure timely assessment
c. Accurate diagnosis and prognosis which deliver realistic and achievable outcomes
d. Competent staff working effectively across boundaries to co-ordinate care
e. Agreed standards and tools for assessment
f. Clear communication with patients/users of services and their carers/relatives

2.11.2 Older people in particular may present with a range of physical, emotional and environmental problems. A programme of health visiting for the assessment of health needs can be used to help prevent potential problems and promote the patient's independence. A health visiting assessment should include assessment of physical, psychological, social and environmental needs for possible referral.

2.11.3 It is important that assessment of an older person should always be holistic and multi-disciplinary, including input from a geriatrician or at least from an experienced general practitioner with a special interest in the care of older people (e.g. Diploma in Geriatric Medicine). This need is met in some areas by community assessment rehabilitation teams (CARTs) led by a consultant geriatrician. CARTSs need to be located in a hospital and form an integral part of the hospital service. The initial decision on the type and purpose of the assessment is crucial for the subsequent delivery of effective care.

2.11.4 There is a range of alternative approaches to individual patient needs assessments, which fall into the following broad categories.

a. Individual clinical assessment by medical practitioners and other health professionals[21]. This assessment may lead to further specialist assessments or for assessments for social care
b. Individual needs assessment for social care. Social service departments assess the individual's needs for personal social services that apply mainly to older people, the mentally ill and those with learning disabilities, those with physical disability, the chronically sick and those with sensory impairment
c. Health screening, most notably annual health assessment of over 75 year olds, available on request from general practitioners. The general practitioner should offer a surgery consultation or home visit by the district nurse to housebound patients. The general assessment should include the patient's physical and mental condition and social environment[22]
d. Specialist assessment such as that undertaken by a physiotherapist, speech and language therapist or occupational therapist. Each of these professions have standards that apply to their assessment procedure
e. Multi-disciplinary assessments for patients with a range of health needs. The multi-disciplinary assessment may be done by a single member of the multi-disciplinary team or a member of each of the different disciplines involved. A nominated key worker should co-ordinate the assessments and subsequent care plan, to avoid the patient and carer repeatedly having to provide the same information. The assessments should all take place within an agreed time-span. Patients requiring a multi-disciplinary assessment may also require a full needs assessment from social services. The resulting care plan should be

jointly decided by the professionals involved, with a key worker responsible for seeing their targets are met

2.11.5   The working group emphasises the importance of establishing generic assessment and care planning/delivery documentation tools (i.e. across services) to assist in the provision of an integrated service to patients. The assessment process should identify the patient's problems and the extent to which needs requiring support may arise. Some needs, particularly where there is a cognitive problem, may be unpredictable[23]. The assessment and resulting care plan should recognise the extent of predictable and potentially unpredictable support needed.

2.11.6   Patients should be initially seen within 5 working days of referral for assessments other than for routine screening purposes. Local agreements covering assessments should include agreed timings.

2.11.7   All community NHS staff must ensure that the patient's general practitioner is informed of the findings of their assessment, and that this information is entered on the patient's records, including those held by the patient.

2.11.8   Eligibility criteria for community health services that relate assessment and treatment to dependency levels[1] developed jointly by the health authority and Trust can enable regular monitoring and assist decisions on the provision of services.

2.11.9   Work carried out on a needs assessment of older people in one particular health authority area[22] has indicated the importance of assessing the prevalence of disease and disability amongst this client group on a population basis to enable more accurate individual needs assessments and the appropriate allocation of resources.

2.12   CARE PLANNING

2.12.1   The patient care plan is derived from the results of assessment. In order to achieve good practice in assessment and care planning, effective communication between agencies and staff as well as with the patients and carers is required. Clear care plans, jointly agreed and accessible to all parties should be formulated. The aim is to ensure that the patient receives the individual care that is needed. Implementation of the care plan should commence within a maximum of 10 working days of being agreed, although there may be specific aspects requiring more rapid action. These should be stipulated.

2.12.2   A care plan for individual patients may be relatively simple or involve a range of professionals and agencies, depending on the outcome of the assessment. The use of professional 'jargon' or terminology not easily understood by those outside a particular discipline should be avoided. The patient and/or carer must be fully involved in the formulation of the care plan. A clear understanding of the treatment and objective of the care plan is essential for a successful outcome.

2.12.3   Whilst the assessment of a carer's needs is a local authority responsibility (see 4.8) the carer's needs will require consideration in the development of the care plan. Both health and other professionals should be ready to advise the carer on obtaining a separate assessment.

2.12.4   The care plan should be reviewed at least every four months, or following a major change in the patient's health or social circumstances.

2.12.5   In some cases, there may be a series of care plans for an individual patient. In this situation it is essential that there should be no conflict between plans, and that each plan should be working towards the same objective and follow the review pattern outlined in 2.12.4.

BOX 8

> **Care planning should include consideration of:**
>
> **a.** Medical treatment - history; current treatment programme; prognosis
> **b.** Psychological state of patient, e.g. fear of falling, fear of becoming forgetful, depression
> **c.** Cognitive and sensory state
> **d.** Home environment
> **e.** Social support networks
> **f.** Provision of equipment including adaptations to the home and personal equipment[4],[6]
> **g.** Communication status including sight and hearing
> **h.** Medication needs
> **i.** Carers needs[25] Under the Carer Recognition and Services Act 1995 carers are entitled to an independent assessment of their needs
> **j.** Welfare benefits advice where appropriate
> **k.** Cultural and religious needs
> **l.** Specific standardised assessments and treatment or intervention by health professionals

The following procedure should be followed in developing the care plan.

BOX 9

> **Each care plan must:**
>
> **a.** Be recorded in writing, signed and dated
> **b.** Be agreed with the patient and/or carer with regard to both short term and long term goals
> **c.** Detail the responsibilities of individuals and agencies
> **d.** Provide a timescale for the achievement of targets
> **e.** Provide contact names and numbers
> **f.** Be sent to everyone concerned including the patient and/or carer unless requested not to by patient, or in cases of suspected abuse
> **g.** Be subject to periodic review

2.13   **PATIENT HELD RECORDS**

2.13.1   A number of community health services and PHCTs have introduced patient held records. This is particularly useful in cases where a number of different professionals may be involved in providing treatment and care. Each time the patient is seen, an entry is made in the record held by the patient. In this way each professional treating the patient has up-to-date information on the status of the patient's overall care management, and the patient is kept fully informed of the care and treatment plans of all professional groups involved.

2.13.2   The introduction of patient held records must be with the agreement of the patient and carer, and the willing participation of all members of the PHCT. If agreement is not reached patient records should be held at an agreed central location, accessible to all the professionals involved.

2.14   **CARE MANAGEMENT**

2.14.1   The effective management of community based care relies on a collaborative approach at managerial and staff levels. The nominated care manager or care co-ordinator is responsible for co-ordinating the service provided under the jointly agreed care plan. Generally the care manager will be from either health or social services depending whether the predominant need is medical or social.

The intention of the care management system is to provide a co-ordinated and flexible response to the needs of the patient. In other words the provision of services should be needs led.

2.14.2   By the nature of their task health service care managers may often need to contact other agencies outside the health setting. They will need to understand the local eligibility criteria being used by social services departments and to familiarise themselves with the costing of a package of care. Multi-disciplinary training may promote more effective joint working between agencies. Inter-disciplinary training should aim to improve collaboration across professions.

2.15   **RISK MANAGEMENT**

2.15.1   The purpose of risk management is to ensure a safe environment for staff, patients and carers, and to enhance the quality of care, thereby also minimising the financial liabilities of the provider organisation. In the case of community services the sites where care is given can range from hospital to the patient's own home. This diversity makes it essential that staff are personally aware of the reporting procedure on risk management issues[26].

2.15.2   The work of all staff working in the community should be covered by risk management policies. These policies should cover three key aspects, namely staff (2.15.3), patients (2.15.6) and the environment (2.15.7).

2.15.3   The Health and Safety at Work Act 1974 applies to all forms of work activity regardless of location. The employer, therefore, has a duty to maintain a safe system of work. This duty extends to staff employed by agencies under contract to health or social services.

2.15.4   The following features should be included in the health and safety policy drawn up and applied to community health or social service.

BOX 10

Aspects to be covered by health and safety policy:

a. Organisational arrangements for implementing the policy, including identification of the location of operational responsibility
b. Maintenance of equipment
c. Safe use, storage and transport of potentially dangerous substances and articles, and their disposal as required by the Control of Pollution (special waste) Regulations. 1980, and Amendments, and COSHH Regulations. 1994
d. Procedures for reporting potential hazards to the responsible manager
e. Procedures for reporting accidents and occupational-related diseases
f. Provision of information, and a training programme, which must include clinical risk management; infection control; responding to violent or aggressive incidents; moving and handling; immediate response to complaints and knowledge of the procedure

---

2.15.5   The following specific measures are recommended for community based staff:

a. Staff should leave a diary of planned visits for each day at their base
b. There should be a guidance protocol addressing safe and secure practice for staff working after 6.00 p.m.
c. Arrangements should be in place for contacting staff on duty (for instance through bleeps, mobile phones or car radio)
d. Provision of suitable lifting and handling equipment must be available wherever and whenever necessary, as assessed by the nurse, physiotherapist or occupational therapist. An agreement between health and social services on the provision of equipment in the community should enable allocation of equipment as needed and avoid bureaucratic delays.

2.15.6   Professional staff have a duty of care to patients which, particularly when they are being treated in their own home, includes advising patients and their carers on safety measures in the home. The essential requirements for patients are shown in box 11 overleaf.

2.15.7   All NHS premises must be kept as clean and safe as possible for staff, patients and visitors. A designated manager must be responsible for ensuring that areas are kept safe from hazards, particularly clinic and waiting areas. This includes operating a system for reporting potential hazards to the responsible manager.

2.15.8   Community staff may experience difficulties in relation to hygiene and infection control through lack of suitable hand washing facilities or inadequate food storage[27]. Training in infection control procedures should include advice on dealing with such problems.

BOX 11

> **Aspects relating to patient safety and welfare in which staff are expected to be competent:**
>
> **a.** Patients being treated in their own homes should receive a full risk assessment which covers patient movement and handling, and level of dependency (including mental capacity)
> **b.** Equipment provided must be safe and in working order and regularly maintained
> **c.** Staff visiting patients should be updated regularly in first aid, and taking emergency action
> **d.** Staff should be alert to signs of elder abuse and aware of guidance on what action to take if abuse is suspected (see also 5.6)

2.15.9   Patients and/or carers receiving home visits should be informed verbally and at the assessment stage of hazards, such as worn carpets, loose wiring and inadequate lighting that could cause accidents in the home. This information should be confirmed in writing to the patient and shared with other agencies involved in the care of the patient.

2.16   TRAINING

2.16.1   Training is important for a number of aspects of community based care and must be provided for community based health staff in the following areas:

   a. Risk management, including safe moving and handling (see Box 12 below)
   b. Clear knowledge of procedures and guidelines for home visits
   c. Understanding of the assessment model being used
   d. Instruction on advice to carers

2.16.2   The UKCC recommends that all practitioners working with older people should receive induction and preparation for their work[28]. In addition all staff must receive induction training which includes the management of risk. As part of their induction, staff need to be introduced to their terms and conditions of employment, the structure of their organisation, the adopted management style, and how supervision is exercised[29]. Box 12 lists areas that must be covered in the induction programme and also form a part of continuing training.

BOX 12

> **As part of their induction and continuing education, all staff must receive training on:**
>
> **a.** First Aid
> **b.** Health and Safety
> **c.** Infection control
> **d.** Emergency action e.g. cardiopulmonary resuscitation
> **e.** Moving and handling
> **f.** Recognition of signs of elder abuse (see also section 5.6)

2.16.3   The working group recommends as best practice that specific training in moving and handling should be jointly organised by health and social services as a means of encouraging a co-ordinated approach to patient care.

2.16.4   Training programmes need to be multi-disciplinary. Together with the associated guidance and procedures, training programmes must be reviewed and updated annually. However multi-disciplinary training does not exclude the need for continual professional updating of skills and ideas.

2.16.5   Records of attendance at training courses (covering at least 12 months) must be kept for each member of staff.

2.17   COMMUNITY CLINICS

2.17.1   Standards for the commissioning of outpatient services in community clinics and in community hospitals are given in the report on service standards for outpatient services[30]. These stipulate that:

   a. Only services that are within the ability of the community clinic or community hospital to deliver are purchased. The provider should have an applied policy in place which sets out the services offered, and the criteria for referral to acute hospital facilities
   b. Value for money is being achieved for patients in rural and town areas, and community hospitals are not being disadvantaged by resources being used to provide community outpatient services
   c. Patients within the catchment area of community hospitals or community clinics and who need the services of outpatient services at an acute general hospital are being appropriately referred. Regular audits (annually) of referrals should take place to see that this happens (see (b) above)
   d. The same standards of time keeping, community information, confidentiality, and as far as possible of the environment, apply to community hospitals or community clinics as apply to outpatient facilities and services provided by acute hospitals.

2.17.2   It is important that clinics to be accessed by older people should be in areas that are easy to locate, clearly signposted and well lit after dark. The clinic should be on ground level or have lift access with adjacent car parking facilities. Environmental requirements for NHS facilities are provided in the service standards report Focus on Patients[31]. The following points taken from that report are particularly relevant for clinic and outpatient department services to older people:

   a. Parking, transport and access including access arrangements for people with disabilities
   b. Waiting areas with chairs of varying heights and with arm rests
   c. Access to a telephone
   d. Toilet and washing facilities

2.17.3   Referral to the clinic should include the outcome of an assessment of the patient's transport needs. Providers are advised to consult the HSA report on patient transport services for standards in this area[32].

2.17.4   Clinics based in the community or at community hospitals should have a designated manager responsible for ensuring that the standards of information given, confidentiality and environmental safety are the same as those which apply to acute hospital outpatient services[30].

2.17.5   Community hospitals or clinics should work to a written statement which describes the services offered and the procedure for referral to acute hospital treatment if required.

2.17.6   The provision of a range of therapeutic services in one place presents an opportunity for health promotion work to help maintain the independence of an older person, particularly if an actively multi-disciplinary approach is adopted to deal with problems - potential or otherwise.

2.18   HEALTH PROMOTION

2.18.1   The value of promoting a healthy lifestyle for older people, and potentially prolonging their independence, is gaining more recognition. Important elements of a health promotion strategy for older people are the prevention and reduction of physical and mental illness.

2.18.2   In the field of prevention, multi-dimensional assessments of older people which include blood pressure, vision, hearing, diet, locomotion and iatrogenic disease may assist in reducing drug usage and hospital admissions. Such assessments can be undertaken by the health visitor.

2.18.3   The reduction of accidents is a Government target in Our Healthier Nation[33], and advice on potential hazards in the home, as well as regular checks of the patient's vision and balance, and for the side effects of medication, may avert serious falls in older people. Studies undertaken by the Health Education Authority[34] have identified the need for local accident prevention strategies specifically targeted at older people. District nurses and health visitors should be alert to the opportunities of advising older people on safety.

2.18.4   Opportunities for general practitioners to make a contribution in the field of prevention of physical and mental illness are available through adoption of the following strategies:

BOX 13

Suggested preventive strategies in primary care
a. Health checks for the over 75 year olds
b. Influenza vaccinations
c. Use of aspirin to minimise the risk of stroke
d. Prescribing exercise and measures to avoid osteoporosis
e. Liaison with health visitors on preventative strategies
f. Liaison with the local authority on social care, housing and transport issues
g. The management of elevated blood pressure
h. Advise on smoking cessation and alcohol
i. Advice on healthy diet consumption
j. Measures to prevent falls

2.18.5   General practices and community health services should have available for their patients information and advice on diet, exercise, smoking, alcohol, depression, sexual health, bereavement and other issues that may impact on the well-being of patients. Local groups providing classes and advice should also be publicised.

2.18.6   Information on the uptake of health promotion and accident prevention services should be undertaken. Audit and evaluation may be required on a long-term basis if significant improvements to outcomes are to be obtained.

3 Hospital based services

The standards in this section relate to the care and treatment of older people in hospital. It is important for those working in the acute sector to be alert to the probability of older people presenting with non-specific conditions and multiple pathology. They may have functional and social problems that impact on their medical condition and mental state.

3.1   ATTENDANCE AT A&E

The HSA report on Standards for A&E Services[5] recommends that patients aged 75 years and over should be given priority in their triage category. The A&E department should have target times for assessment of these patients.

3.1.1   A protocol agreed between the A&E department and the department of geriatric medi-cine/medical directorate must provide for a physician, preferably one specialising in geriatric medicine (or undergoing specialist training in it, i.e. a registrar) to attend elderly patients in the A&E department within 30 minutes of request or 10 minutes in urgent cases[35].

3.1.2   The A&E department should have written protocols, agreed with the department of elderly medicine, covering management of commonly presenting conditions in older people, such as falls, confusion, dizziness.

3.1.3   If a patient is brought in by ambulance a report from the paramedics should be recorded before they leave.

3.1.4   The home circumstances of the older person should be ascertained at triage to ensure that arrangements are made to care for any dependent relative. Triage should also identify whether an interpreter is needed, or if the patient has a hearing and/or visual impairment.

3.1.5   Access to a multi-disciplinary team must be available for a more detailed assessment, if indicated by screening. There should be access to occupational therapy for equipment or aids that could enable a return home rather than admission.

3.1.6   Specialist nursing advice on the elderly must be available to A&E as a minimum standard. The best practice standard is for a specialist nurse to be attached to the A&E department.

3.1.7   The general practitioner must be informed in writing (or if initially by telephone, then con-firmed in writing) within 24 hours of the attendance at the A&E department of any individual patient over 75 years on their list. If the patient is discharged, the general practi-tioner should be informed by telephone within one working day (or within 48 hours at the weekend). The information given must include plans made for follow-up. The general prac-titioner must also be informed by telephone of the death of a patient on his/her list within one working day (or 48 hours at the weekend).

3.1.8   A district liaison nurse or health visitor should be attached to the A&E department with the specific responsibility of ensuring that the general practitioner is informed of the attendance of elderly patients and that requested follow up care takes place. Normally older patients should not be discharged at weekends, Bank holidays or after 5.00 p.m. unless the liaison nurse is satisfied that adequate home arrangements are in place and the patient and carer agree.

3.1.9   The British Geriatrics Society recommend that local A&E policies and procedures should also cover:

  a. Referral for urgent clinic or day hospital assessment
  b. Referral for community based rehabilitation
  c. Referral for urgent residential care

3.1.10   Protocols covering the discharge home of older people from A&E, and referral of patients for urgent social care, should be agreed with local social services.

3.1.11   All recumbent elderly patients must be placed on pressure relieving mattresses (preferably on beds not trolleys) through their stay in A&E.

3.2   ADMISSION FROM A&E

3.2.1   Patients should wait no longer than 2 hours from the time of the decision to admit to the ward and no more than a total of 3 hours from their initial arrival to admission[5].

3.2.2   The decision to admit patients in need of multi-disciplinary geriatric care should be based on local criteria established with the department of geriatric medicine. A&E should be aware of the criteria. The time taken from the decision to admit the patient and actually reaching the ward should be regularly monitored.

3.2.3   All accident and emergency departments should work to a written procedure designed to ensure the safety of older patients on beds or trolleys.

3.3   AGREED ADMISSIONS

3.3.1   When agreement has been reached with a general practitioner to admit an elderly patient electively, this should not be cancelled by the proposed admitting facility unless the circumstances are exceptional. When a cancellation is unavoidable, the general practitioner must be informed on the same day as the decision to cancel. A new date for admission must be agreed at the same time.

3.3.2   Patients for whom admission to hospital is being arranged must be notified of the date and time; preparative requirements; personal possessions to take; notice of organisational arrangements, which must include whether the ward is single or mixed sex, and whether there are segregated washing and toilet facilities (see also 3.9).

3.4   CARE OF OLDER PEOPLE ON THE WARD

3.4.1   A clear statement of the patient's current (active) and previous (inactive) medical and physical problems should be present in the patient's notes. The medical notes of older persons admitted to hospital as emergency inpatients must be retrieved from medical records and available to medical staff within two hours of the patient's admission. In non-emergency cases the medical records must be available within 24 hours. Previous X-rays must be made available within 12 hours of admission at the latest.

3.4.2   The admissions clerk/nurse should include a statement of the patient's social circumstances in the patient's notes. This should include whether the patient has carer responsibilities at home, pets left at home and if there is a nominated key holder. The name of the person that the patient wishes to be involved for the purpose of planning future care or because of a change in his/her condition, and whether he/she has made a living will, should also be recorded.

3.4.3   Procedures should be in place to ensure that patients receive essential information on their arrival at the ward. If the patient is not well enough to comprehend, the relative/carer, if present, should be given the information listed in Box 14. All nurses have a responsibility to inform patients of the services available within the hospital.

BOX 14

> **Information to be given to the patient on arrival on the ward[31]:**
>
> **a.** Name of the ward
> **b.** How the ward/inpatient facility is structured, procedures, visiting times etc.
> **c.** Name of the ward manager/senior nurse
> **d.** Name of the patient's named nurse and their substitute (when off duty or not available)
> **e.** Names of permanent ward staff, including the advice that nursing, ancillary and student nurse names are available on the ward notice board
> **f.** Information on the medical staff including the name of the consultant, senior house officer, etc.
> **g.** Arrangements for meals and other eating facilities (see also 3.10)
> **h.** Arrangements for visiting, contacting and being contacted by friends and relatives
> **i.** Other information relevant to their stay in hospital (e.g. expected day/time of operation)
> **j.** Procedure for complaints, obtaining a patient advocate

3.4.4   The named nurse is responsible for ensuring that this information (Box 14) reaches the patient and for referring the patient to other services. The ward manager has overall responsibility for ensuring that the patient receives any services requested e.g. social worker, chaplain, nutritional advice, complaints officer, hairdresser or volunteer services.

3.4.5   A nursing assessment must be commenced on admission, and should form the basis for immediate care in conjunction with the multi-disciplinary team. Areas listed in Box 15 need to be addressed using a systematic framework.

BOX 15

Topics which must be addressed by the nurse conducting initial patient assessment on admission:

a. Vision
b. Hearing
c. Mobility and balance (feet, joints/gait)
d. Nutritional status, body mass index
e. Ability to eat or swallow
f. Teeth/dentures
g. Appetite
h. Medication prior to admission
i. Blood pressure and pulse
j. Mental health - cognition
k. Pressure sore risk
l. Bladder and bowel function
m. Risk of falling
n. Spiritual issues, including recent bereavement
o. Home environment and social support

3.4.6   A clear written protocol should be available setting out the care pathway for older people newly admitted to the ward. This should include screening and assessment by medical staff.

3.4.7   Initial nursing and medical assessments provide essential baseline information prior to referral for multi-disciplinary assessment.

There is a growing evidence of the value in both medical and cost-effective terms, of Comprehensive Geriatric Assessment. The greatest value appears to be found in inpatient geriatric evaluation units, which have often been dissipated in the rush towards integration of acute medical services. The use of such assessment models should be considered for both hospital and community based clients/patients/consumers presenting with predominant health or social needs[36,37].

An initial multi-disciplinary assessment should therefore cover social, functional and environmental as well as medical needs. This reflects the principle that an early, thorough assessment and identification of potential problems could avoid difficulties in discharge planning. Liaison with community health services on patients known to them, may prevent unnecessary assessments and assist effective care planning.

3.4.8   The named nurse has the responsibility of co-ordinating this multi-disciplinary assessment. Initial multi-disciplinary assessment should include a statement of the patient's capabilities before admission. Other aspects that should be included in this initial assessment are given in Box 16.

BOX 16

The following aspects should be included in an initial multi-disciplinary assessment:

a. Communication status including sight/hearing

b. Nutritional needs

c. Continence

d. Pressure sores (including a risk assessment using a recognised standardised tool e.g. Waterlow score)

e. Activities of daily living (ADL) measurement, using a standard scale e.g. Barthel score

f. Assessment of risk of falling

g. Cognitive assessment using a standard scale e.g. Abbreviated Mental Test score

---

3.4.9   A consultant-led multi-disciplinary review following treatment of immediate problems should be undertaken weekly. Medically led ward rounds should be twice weekly on acute wards and at least once a week on rehabilitation wards or in community hospitals.

3.4.10   Consultant-led multi-disciplinary review meetings should be held on the ward, at least once a week rather than the team placing its reliance on collaborative documentation alone.

3.4.11   Continuity of care is essential. Movement of patients between wards should be based on the individual patient's clinical need and not on organisational convenience.

3.5   **ACCESS TO OTHER INVESTIGATIONS**

3.5.1   Older people must have equal rights with all other patients to access investigations to confirm diagnosis and to ascertain appropriateness of the proposed treatment where this is judged necessary by the doctor. Investigations and management which must be equitably accessible to older patients will include cardiological investigations, access to CCU, radiology CT/MRI scans and access to specialist nursing services. Procedures should be in place for monitoring appropriate referral to and uptake of these services for patients aged 75 years and above, including the timing of uptake.

3.6   **PAIN MANAGEMENT**

Detailed standards for pain management are to be published in the HSA report Standards for Anaesthetic Services currently in preparation. The purpose of this section is to highlight particular aspects of pain management relevant to older people.

Pain and distress may be experienced in several dimensions, involving states of physiological, psychological, social and spiritual well-being[38]. Each of these has special significance for older people. For instance, the older person may already have diminished functional ability, be suffering psychological distress and enjoy a limited social life. Where possible the management of pain in older people should go beyond pharmacological intervention. A holistic approach is particularly suitable for adoption by community services (see 3.6.6).

3.6.1 Possible barriers to effective pain management for older people may be:

  a. The patient believes everything possible is being done and is reluctant to complain of pain or distress
  b. The health care team believes older patients cannot tolerate opioids, and that pain perception decreases with age
  c. The patient and his/her carers fear addiction or side effects, and consider pain to be an inevitable consequence of surgery
  d. The health care team fail to address other than physical symptoms

3.6.2 The most effective post-operative pain management plan should be based on 'balanced analgesia' thereby reducing any potential side-effects from a single agent. In the case of operations known to be particularly painful, such as certain orthopaedic procedures, pre-emptive analgesia such as nerve block may be very effective.

3.6.3 The following protocol is recommended for the management of post-operative pain in older patients.

BOX 17

> **Protocol for management of pain should include:**
>
>   a. Assessment of pain using a pain rating scale every 1-2 hours during the first 24 hours
>   b. Assessment thereafter every 2-4 hours
>   c. Pain flow chart and medication record must be kept

3.6.4 Management of cancer pain should follow the WHO concept of using oral medication wherever possible, with continuous, round the clock administration. Reasons for using alternative methods will include evidence of poor pain control, swallowing problems, and a dysfunctional gastrointestinal system.

3.6.5 There should be close co-operation between the pain management service, the general practitioner, and Macmillan nurses (if involved), in the administration and review of pain relief for patients at home.

3.6.6 Studies undertaken in the United States of America and referred to by Ferrell[38] suggest that a combination of pharmacological and other methods yield the most effective pain relief. The use of non-drug pain relief methods should be in addition to drug treatment and should generally be started after adequate drug treatment has been established.

3.6.7 The following principles should be followed when establishing a programme for the use of non-drug interventions.

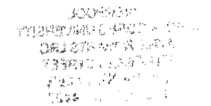

BOX 18

Non-drug methods of pain management:
a. Emphasise non-drug intervention as an addition to (not replacement of) drug therapy
b. Offer a variety of pain relief methods and evaluate their effectiveness
c. Provide written information to accompany verbal instructions
d. Incorporate the patient's values and beliefs in the treatment programme
e. Involve carers to reduce any sense of helplessness on their part

3.7   REFERRAL TO THERAPIES

3.7.1   The adopted referral pathway to the therapies should be clearly understood by ward staff, and form part of the written induction material. Requirements may vary between hospitals and for different disciplines within the same hospital. Physiotherapists may prioritise within a blanket system of referrals for instance, whilst other therapies, such as speech and language therapy, may require and respond to individual written referral letters.

3.7.2   Referral to therapies should include an agreed maximum time limit within which a referral should be actioned.

3.7.3   Each therapy team should include a professional with at least one year's experience in the care of older people and/or a recognised qualification in the care of older people.

3.8   STAFFING

3.8.1   Recruitment difficulties have inevitably led to an increasing reliance on the use of agency nurses. The group recommends that Trusts should plan for a minimum level of 75% permanent staff in nursing. This should enable patients to experience continuity of care whilst in hospital. The best practice standard would be for 90% of nurses to be on substantive contracts. The senior nurse in clinical areas dedicated to the care of older patients should hold a relevant post-graduate nursing diploma/or degree.

3.8.2   The clinical skill mix on acute geriatric medical wards should be the same as that on general medical wards. All clinical staff should receive training in the care of older people, demonstrated by a programme of continual professional development and in-service training made available to all. Continuous professional development requires a formal mechanism of staff appraisal. The British Geriatric Society (BGS) recommends that all doctors involved in the medical management of acutely ill older patients should have post-graduate training in geriatric medicine[39]. Minimum qualifications and required experience for posts should appear on all medical job descriptions.

3.9   WARD FACILITIES

3.9.1   Patients must be informed if it is proposed that their care will be given on a mixed sex ward. EL(97)3. The Patient's Charter: Privacy and Dignity and the Provision of Single Sex Accommodation, requires all Trusts to offer accommodation on single-sex wards. This may not always be an immediate possibility in all settings, for instance in older buildings. Intensive care and coronary care units with high tech equipment and admission wards are exempt. All Trusts, however, should have plans to achieve this objective within a specified period. It is essential, unless special equipment is being used, that separate toilet and washing facilities for men and women, within easy reach of their beds, are available and clearly marked[40].

3.9.2 Facilities on the ward should include adequate space around beds to accommodate hoists and pressure relief equipment. Wards should have anti-slip flooring. Beds must have call bells and induction loop facilities.

3.9.3 In principle, restraint should only be used as a final resort and for a short time only. A policy on patient handling and the use of restraint should be in place. This policy should outline procedures for monitoring and reviewing the type and frequency of restraints used[(10)]. Restraint should only be applied with the agreement of a senior nurse and a senior doctor trained in geriatric medicine. The reasons for restraint must be documented[41], together with a risk assessment of the circumstances leading to the restraint.

3.9.4 A separate room should be available for private interviewing.

3.9.5 Patients should have individual lockers for their personal effects, including facilities for dentures and clothes. Older patients should be encouraged to dress in day time clothes and wear safe footwear, once the acute phase of their stay is over. Large faced clocks on the ward aid orientation to day/night and a resumption of normal life.

3.9.6 A written Trust protocol on the safe keeping of valuables and belongings, including clothes, must be kept on the ward, known to and observed by staff and made known to patients and carers.

3.9.7 The movement of elderly patients between wards and clinical teams should be minimised in order to prevent disorientation of the patient, family anxiety, discontinuity of care, and delay in effective discharge planning. Systems should be in place to track older patients through departments and wards. The operation of these systems and the incidence of movement should be audited.

3.10 NUTRITION

3.10.1 Many older people may have been having inadequate nutrition prior to their hospital admission. It is therefore important that the nutritional status of each patient is assessed in accordance with hospital guidelines prepared with input from the dietetics service. It is recommended that at least one nurse on each ward has a specific interest in nutrition[42]. Advice may be needed from the Trust's dietician/nutrition support service, and/or a referral made to the speech and language therapist for swallowing problems. Advice from the dietician on patients identified as being at nutritional risk should be available within 24 hours.

3.10.2 Protocols for the provision of parenteral nutrition for very ill older patients should be adopted and observed. All Trusts must have and observe a written local protocol governing the insertion of gastronomy (PEG) tubes, and the management of this intervention should be subject to routine clinical audit.

3.10.3   Older people are generally at risk of under nutrition and dehydration, and this risk is increased by hospital admission. Provision of nutritious and attractive meals for patients during their stay in hospital is an important aid to recovery. The HSA report Focus on Patients recommends that the maximum time from the last main meal at night to breakfast the following day should not exceed 14 hours. However there is evidence that 14 hours is too long for older people to be without food[42]. The availability of snacks on the ward can avoid this difficulty.

3.10.4   The hospital menu should cater for the preferences and nutritional needs of older people. Food suitable to meet patients' religious and cultural preferences should also be provided.

3.10.5   Particular attention to acutely confused patients is needed to encourage them to eat and drink. This can be aided by dietary supplements, such as nutritious drinks available on the ward. Arrangements should be made, possibly with visitors, to assist patients unable to feed themselves, at meal times.

3.10.6   Ensuring that their patients are fed is a core function of the care nurses are expected to provide to their patients[43]. General nutrition and the techniques of nutritional support should be included in the continuing education of all nursing and medical staff caring for older patients. All departments of geriatric medicine should ensure that all wards/units where their patients are lodged have and apply a written operational policy designed to ensure their patients are fed. The policy will identify nursing staff responsible for its practical implementation and include procedural notes and guidelines designed to ensure its delivery.

3.10.7   Patients identified on admission as having swallowing difficulties should be assessed by a speech and language therapist within at least two working days of receipt of the referral.

3.11   OUTPATIENT SERVICES

The initial referral to an outpatient clinic is generally for a specialist assessment. Detailed standards for outpatient clinics are given in the Health Services Accreditation report on Standards for Outpatient Services[30].

3.11.1   National standards on waiting times for a first appointment stipulate that nine out of ten people can expect to be seen within thirteen weeks and everyone can expect to be seen within 26 weeks. However, recognising that relatively minor problems in older patients can deteriorate quickly, it is recommended that all new referrals of older people should expect to be seen within four weeks, and all urgent referrals be seen within one week.

3.11.2   Notification of the appointment must include date, time, exact location and whether transport is being organised. The information should be clearly laid out and include a contact number for the patient or carer to use. Visual impairment or cognitive difficulties should be considered when making appointments e.g. by using large print letters on forms.

3.11.3   A written reminder or telephone call nearer to the appointment date may reduce the DNA (did not attend) rate. Transport arrangements, particularly for older patients, can be checked with the patient/carer on this occasion.

3.11.4   If the patient is being referred from their outpatient clinic to another consultant, or for treatment (such as physiotherapy), the doctor and clinic nurse should seek to ensure that the patient and/or carer understands what is proposed. The general practitioner must be informed of this further referral within one week.

3.11.5   No hospital investigations should be refused to an older patient on the grounds of old age alone.

3.11.6   Facilities of particular importance to older people include:

a. Wheelchairs and porters available to take patients between hospital areas
b. Chairs of varying height in the waiting area (with/without arms)
c. Refreshments, including tea and coffee, available within or close by the waiting area
d. Toilet facilities, including provision for the disabled, close by the waiting area
e. Services available for patients with visual or hearing difficulties

3.11.7   Staff caring for older patients should have experience of their needs and should have access to in-house training and continuing external education.

3.12   **DAY HOSPITAL CARE**

Day hospital care offers a specialist day facility for outpatients, run by an NHS Trust. In the case of an acute Trust it will often form part of the service provided by the hospital's department of geriatric medicine. Day hospitals run by community Trusts need to ensure regular consultant geriatrician input to the day hospital service, perhaps on a sessional basis.

3.12.1   There should be clear definition of the functions and aims of the day hospital. Day hospitals provide medical, rehabilitative and therapeutic services. The function of day hospitals is not to provide social care (which is provided by day care centres). The level of dependency exhibited by older patients attending day hospital may be significant and service providers must anticipate this and plan appropriate levels of response[24].

3.12.2   There should be arrangements for a daily visit from a doctor from the Department of Geriatric Medicine to visit the day hospital.

3.12.3   The objectives of attendance at the day hospital should be clearly defined and are likely to cover the functions listed in Box 19.

BOX 19

Main functions of geriatric day hospitals:

a. Medical and multi-disciplinary assessment
b. Rehabilitation
c. Maintenance of functional ability/independence
d. Provision of medical and nursing procedures
e. Promotion of personal hygiene
f. A base for the community assessment rehabilitation team (CART)

3.12.4   There should be access to a range of medical and paramedical staff. This is often facilitated by the location of the day hospital at a general hospital site.

3.12.5   The range of expertise to be available is listed in Box 20.

BOX 20

Staff whose services should be available in the day hospital:

a. Consultant geriatrician
b. Nursing staff
c. Physiotherapist
d. OT
e. Speech and language therapist
f. Social worker

Referrals from the day hospital may be made to the following staff whose services may be provided either on site or elsewhere:

g. Physicians from other specialities
h. Psychogeriatrician
i. Psychologist
j. Continence adviser
k. Dietician
l. Chiropodist
m. Other specialist nurses
n. Dentist
o. Optician
p. ENT/audiology
q. Surgical appliances
r. General practitioner

3.12.6   Referral to the day hospital may follow on discharge from hospital (as an inpatient) or come from the general practitioner, district nurse, or consultant-led team, e.g. psychiatry for the elderly. Patients discharged from hospital and referred to the day hospital should not be required to wait for an appointment. Urgent referrals should be seen within two working days and the remainder within one week. Day hospitals should not have waiting lists.

Day hospital care plans should include specific goals for the patient to achieve. Planned discharge from programmes of day hospital care should be discussed at multi-disciplinary, consultant-led meetings. Planning must involve the patient and (where appropriate) the carer. The general practitioner must be notified of the planned discharge date and of any significant changes in therapy introduced during attendance. Liaison with social services, if required, should also take place prior to discharge (see also 4.7).

3.13 REHABILITATION

3.13.1 Rehabilitation is a crucial aspect in the care of older people. The process may take place in hospital and/or at home, it may be specialised (as for stroke) or more generally focused.

3.13.2 In hospital, patients may expect to be treated and cared for by a multi-disciplinary team which recognises their potential abilities and encourages (rehabilitates) them by means of exercise and other programmes so that they can return to as independent a life as possible.

3.13.3 The British Geriatrics Society (BGS) have identified the different aspects which need to be addressed through rehabilitation. These are listed in Box 21.

BOX 21

Aspects that need to be included in the rehabilitative process:

a. The damaged system
b. Other body systems
c. Psychological attitudes
d. Coping with the immediate environment e.g. clothes
e. Coping with the near environment e.g. housing
f. Coping with the distant environment e.g. shops
g. Social support networks

3.13.4 These different aspects illustrate the central requirement for a multi-disciplinary/multi-agency approach.

3.13.5 Rehabilitation should begin as soon as possible after the onset of acute illness.

3.13.6 Each patient should progress through the following stages: assessment; planning (which should include goal setting); treatment; evaluation; care and finally advice on coping strategies. Standardised measures should be used to assess the patient's progress.

3.13.7 The multiple needs of older people may require lengthier rehabilitation. The multi-disciplinary team should agree that the patients' maximum abilities have been achieved before rehabilitation ceases.

3.13.8 The facilities (beds) provided for the rehabilitation of older inpatients should be located in areas distinct from those offering acute care or care for the terminally ill.

3.13.9   No patient should have their rehabilitation curtailed because of pressure on hospital beds or other external considerations.

3.13.10   Rehabilitation should continue after discharge from hospital. This may, with the patient's agreement, involve his/her family and other carers. Arrangements should be made prior to discharge in conjunction with social services for continuing support and rehabilitation in the community.

3.13.11   Reviews of the care plan should include whether all planned services are being provided. Reviews should include 'simple' as well as 'complex' cases in order to ensure proper targeting of both health and social services provision[44].

3.13.12   Health authorities and local authorities, in partnership with NHS Trusts, are currently (1998) reviewing the provision of recuperation and rehabilitation services for older people. Their review must include an analysis of current and future need as well as an audit of current service provision and an agreed joint plan of service development[20]. In addition, as part of their work on a framework for multi-disciplinary assessment, health and local authorities have also been asked to establish a range of rehabilitation facilities funded by the Special Transitional Grant[19].

3.14   CLINICAL RISK MANAGEMENT

3.14.1   Trusts providing inpatient care for older people should be aware that the achievement in practice of the organisational, procedural and performance standards contained in this report will provide considerable assurance that effective risk management is undertaken by those responsible for the care of the elderly and by their collaborating services. However Trusts will seek to ensure they have, and apply, explicit risk management policies. Health Services Accreditation recognises that the standards for systematic risk management adopted by the Clinical Negligence Scheme for Trusts (CNST) represent an effective organisational framework[45,46].

3.14.2   Departments of geriatric medicine must ensure that along with the critical areas of patient falls, their risk management policy and risk preventing procedures will also address the topics of safe hot water (temperature never to exceed 43°C - NHS Guidelines), infection control (with particular reference to MRSA) and the administration of drugs.

4 Communicating between services

4.1 BACKGROUND

Good communications, whether between services, agencies or members of a multi-disciplinary team, provide the basis for mutual understanding. Incorrect assumptions can lead to inadequate provision or sometimes negligence in patient care. Agencies must have guidance for staff, and ensure that they have a clear understanding of the procedures to be followed in their dealings with other professionals. This is the only way in which the patient's experience of the care they receive will be seamless.

4.2 PRINCIPLES OF COMMUNICATION

The greater number of professionals and agencies involved in the provision of services the greater the risk of failures in communication. Communication methods therefore cannot be left to individual practitioners to decide upon without any guidance, but should be addressed through joint consideration by multi-disciplinary teams and between collaborative agencies.

4.3 COMMUNICATIONS POLICIES

All health services should have a clear written communications policy covering the following:

a. Ensuring communication skills for direct patient contact, including training for obtaining consent for planned procedures (see also the HSA report Focus on Patients)
b. Transfer of up to date clinical information
c. Maintenance of patient records
d. Procedures for inter-departmental and inter-agency communication
e. Confidentiality

4.3.1 Patient records on computer should be protected for confidentiality but also link acute, community (including primary) and social care. A summary should be held by the patient.

4.4 THE GENERAL PRACTITIONER

The general practitioner is central to the patient's experience of the health service. Almost without exception all health care information needs to be fed back to the general practitioner. The line between health and social care needs is becoming increasingly blurred and the general practitioner should be made aware of the involvement of local authority services and other agencies in providing support to his/her patients. In principle then, the information that the general practitioner should receive about his/her patients is now broader and more extensive. Likewise the general practitioner's knowledge of other services and how they can be accessed also needs to be comprehensive and up to date.

4.5 REFERRALS

4.5.1 The general practitioner provides the most regular referral route to other services. The following requirements are recommended by the HSA primary care service standards working group and form the basis for effective referral from the general practitioner, to hospital based or other services.

BOX 22

Minimum requirements for a routine referral letter: **a.** Patient's name and marital status **b.** Date of birth **c.** Address (with postcode) and telephone number **d.** NHS number **e.** Identifying reference (if the patient has been seen by the hospital before) **f.** Presenting complaint and report of general practitioner clinical examination **g.** Treatment already initiated, past medical history and any medication or investigations performed by referring agent and copies of results of investigations **h.** Suggested diagnosis **i.** Social factors including the role of the carer which could influence management **j.** Other needs including domestic circumstances, or other factors which may influence care planning and management e.g. availability of patient, disabilities, transport, religious belief relevant to treatment, need for an interpreter, bilingual advocate **k.** Indication of what response the referrer expects from the clinician referred to

4.5.2   It is also recommended that general practitioners have direct access to consultants and their teams in line with an agreed protocol.

4.5.3   There should also be an established procedure for members of the PHCT to contact other services such as social services, transport, therapists and specialist nursing services for the purpose of referring patients to them. A careful record should be kept of all such communications.

4.6   **RECORD KEEPING**

4.6.1   The recording of all assessments in a shared care record is helpful both for older people and the professionals involved because of the inter-agency and multi-disciplinary nature of their care and treatment.

4.6.2   A copy of the shared care record should always remain with the patient. The record should include essential information on the patient, assessments (including names and contact numbers of those involved) and the clinical and social care plan. Essential aspects to be covered include health, functional status and social support. Information that does not need to be shared by the health care team should not be included.

4.6.3   Patients may need to be reassured of their right to withhold sight of their records from carers, relatives, neighbours and others not professionally involved in their care.

4.7   **COMMUNICATION ON DISCHARGE FROM HOSPITAL**

4.7.1   Hospitals must have a comprehensive discharge planning policy which includes reference to identified categories of patients with particular needs. The policy should emphasise the importance of commencing discharge planning at the time of admission and involving the patient and carer(s).

4.7.2 The general method of communicating notice of discharge is for a short discharge summary to be sent to the patient's general practitioner, followed by a more informative letter. The HSA report on Service Standards for Discharge Care[6] details the information which must be included in the immediate discharge communication. Details appear in Box 23 below.

4.7.3 Some Trusts or departments of geriatric medicine have introduced standardised discharge letters with check lists. The introduction of standardised referral or discharge letters should be by agreement between primary and secondary care clinicians and staff.

BOX 23

Items of information to be included in the immediate discharge communication issued at the point of patient discharge from hospital[6]:

a. General practitioner identification
b. Patient identification
c. Admitting ward (and discharge ward where different), consultant's name, hospital details
d. Dates of admission, discharge, signing off of discharge communication
e. Name and signature of discharging clinician
f. Relevant medical investigations performed
g. Provisional diagnosis of presenting symptoms
h. Treatment(s) given
i. Drugs prescribed on discharge and duration
j. Future medical management including follow-up
k. Outpatient appointment details
l. Where patient discharged to
m. Community care arranged
n. Comments on patient dependency level and functional ability
o. Information given to patient and carer
p. Unresolved matters
q. Indication as to whether more information is to follow
r. The responsible doctor from whom the general practitioner can obtain further information

---

4.7.4 The procedure for linking with community and social services prior to discharge of patients from hospital is often crucially important for older people. Arrangements with hospital based social services staff may vary but assessments by hospital based social services enable support services to be arranged so as to be available on discharge of the patient. The process of assessment should include the patient, carer and relevant hospital and community based professions[44].

4.7.5 Service Standards for Discharge Care (section 9) details a screening procedure to identify those needing a comprehensive community care assessment. Box 24 lists the categories of patient (relevant to older people) whom screening will identify for this assessment.

BOX 24

Significant factors in identifying patients who require community care assessment prior to discharge:

a. Elderly people living alone
b. People returning home to a carer who may have difficulty coping
c. Seriously ill patients who may need to return to hospital
d. Terminally ill patients
e. People with a continuing physical disability and/or who have a learning disability or cognitive impairment
f. People with mental health problems including dementia
g. Homeless people or those in poor housing
h. People with caring responsibilities
i. People suspected of being abused
j. Those unable to return home

4.7.6   The patient's named nurse or the discharge liaison nurse or other designated member of staff, is responsible for requesting a formal community care assessment from social services. The responsible nurse is also in a position to arrange temporary practical support for older people being discharged home.

4.8   **CARERS**

4.8.1   Under the Carers (Recognition and Services) Act, 1995[47] which relates to informal carers, the carer may request the local authority (social services department (SSD)) for an assessment of his/her ability to provide for the relevant person. The results of the assessment must be taken into account in deciding on the provision of community services.

4.8.2   The assessment of the carer is a local authority responsibility, although health professionals may be well placed to make an initial assessment of the stress a carer is under. It should be recognised that the needs of the carer may conflict with those of the person for whom the person is caring. A clearer view of the circumstances may be obtained by the use of different assessors[48]. All agencies should be both ready to advise the carer on how to obtain an assessment, and be prepared to contribute to it.

4.8.3   The need for carers to have adequate information in order to carry out their responsibilities is self-evident. In asking the patient for consent to disclose information to the carer, health professionals should emphasise the importance for the carer to have a clear understanding of the patient's condition and the prognosis, whilst acknowledging the patient's right to refuse to allow disclosure of information. Aspects important to carers are[49]:

a. Medical condition of the patient
b. Chances of improvement
c. Signs of relapse
d. The patient's limitations, including communication, exercise, diet
e. Professional support available
f. Psychological aspects for patient and carer

g. Welfare benefits

h. Respite care

i. Information on support groups

4.8.4   Carers need to be closely involved in the planned discharge of the patient. The nurse responsible needs to ensure that the carer understands and can meet the needs of the patient and receives advice on the use of equipment.

4.8.5   As well as providing the opportunity for rehabilitation and assessment, the provision of respite care is an essential feature of meeting the needs of carers. There should be close liaison between health and social services on the availability of respite care, day care and other support services that will assist the carer.

4.8.6   Guidance issued by the DoH (HSC(98)159)[50] sets the national context for local plans to achieve national priorities in health and social care. A shared lead (i.e. health and social services) includes targeting a range of preventative services for adults, including respite care. Further guidance for an action plan will be issued in early 1999.

4.9   **HOSPITAL AT HOME**

Evidence of the benefits of hospital at home schemes in terms of patient well being, reduced pressure on hospital beds and reduced costs is at present inconclusive. Positive outcomes seem to be related to the presenting condition, with some positive effects on cost and reduced length of time in hospital (relating to specialist rehabilitation for stroke and fractured femur).

4.9.1   It is necessary for the successful introduction of a hospital at home scheme for prior discussions to have taken place with general practitioners leading to agreement over clinical responsibility. District nursing, community physiotherapy and community pharmacy services should all be closely involved in setting up the service.

4.9.2   The support of the relatives and/or informal carers of individual patients eligible for hospital at home management will be needed. They will need advice on the day-to-day management of the patient. The freedom of choice for families being offered the scheme should be emphasised.

4.9.3   The working group recommends that the standards listed in Box 25 should be applied to a hospital at home scheme.

BOX 25

Standards for a hospital at home scheme:

a. There must be clear designation of the clinically responsible person (i.e. consultant or general practitioner)

b. Patient referral should be through the acute services

c. The patient should have a medical and nursing assessment against the criteria for acceptance for hospital at home

d. Close communication must be maintained between the patient's consultant and the general practitioner

e. Experienced occupational therapy and physiotherapy support should be integral to the hospital at home team, and available at short notice

f. Care workers must be trained in the provision of nursing, social, domestic, therapy and medication tasks

g. Close liaison and flexible working is required between the acute unit and the hospital at home scheme team as well as within the hospital at home team

h. Community health services should be involved in the management of the scheme

i. The communication link to social services should be clearly understood by all the professionals involved

j. Arrangements to implement the service for patients assessed as suitable should start immediately

k. There must be immediate access to a hospital bed/or other secondary care facility for patients whose condition deteriorates

l. There must be equal access to investigation and other secondary care facilities for patients managed under a hospital at home scheme as for equivalent patients in hospital

m. Discharge from the hospital at home scheme must be according to clearly set goals

n. Families and carers should be offered choice regarding their level of involvement in care provision at home

5 Maintaining the patient's dignity

5.1 CONSENT

The patient's consent to their clinical management is a basic requirement for the provision of health care. However, this consent must be informed consent, and the patient must have sufficient understandable information to enable a meaningful choice to be made. Permission given under pressure is not consent[51],[10]. An interpreter will be needed for patients with a limited knowledge of English.

5.1.2 Obtaining a signature does not mean that the consent is necessarily valid. The patient must have been told and must fully understand the nature and purpose of the proposed treatment. It is therefore extremely important to have details in the patient notes of the explanation given to the patient when consent was obtained. Consent must be obtained by a health professional experienced in performing the proposed procedure.

5.1.3 Oral consent may be implied (as when the patient allows a physical examination by the doctor) or verbal (for minor investigations or treatments). Like written consent, verbal consent should be recorded in the patient's notes, with relevant details, and signed and dated by the clinician involved.

5.1.4 Written consent should be obtained for any procedure or treatment carrying any substantial risk or side effect[52]. The patient should receive a copy of their signed consent form, and their signed consent, with all relevant details, must also be kept in the patient's notes.

5.1.5 Aspects listed in Box 26 must be covered when obtaining informed patient consent.

BOX 26

> **In order to achieve valid consent, patients must[53]:**
>
> **a.** Be given clear and straightforward information about the proposed treatment by someone experienced in the procedure
> **b.** Be advised about possible alternatives and associated risks
> **c.** Have any questions they may ask answered
> **d.** Be able to withdraw consent

5.1.6 A patient's ability to appreciate the significance of information should be assessed[53]. Older patients with sensory impairment, specific communication problems or if in shock or pain may have difficulty understanding the information given to them. Assessment of the patient's capacity to consent can be helped by inviting him/her to ask questions[10]. Where it is possible, and the patient is in agreement, a close family member or friend can assist at the discussions.

Patients suffering from dementia may be capable of consent or refusal of consent. Each patient's capability for giving consent has to be judged individually in the light of the nature of the decision required and the mental state of the patient at the time[52]. The competence of such patients to understand may also vary over time. Care is needed on selecting appropriate opportunities for raising consent matters[10].

5.1.7   Trust guidance on obtaining consent should include a procedure for action if the patient cannot consent. In such circumstances the doctor should act in the best interests of the patient, following consultation with the nearest relative or friend.

5.2   **CONFIDENTIALITY**

All acute general hospitals and community Trusts must have a written policy safeguarding confidential information and the procedures for disclosure of such information[(31)]. All employees and voluntary staff have a duty of confidence towards patients. The policy should cover circumstances in which disclosure of patient information can or should be made[(53)].

5.2.1   The Caldicott Committee[54] recommends that the transfer of patient identifiable information should have a clearly defined purpose and be justifiable. The report also recommends a model notice for patients, explaining the reasons for passing on information and explaining provisions of the Data Protection Act 1988. Staff involved in processing data must also understand the broad provisions of this Act.

5.2.2   Patients themselves may be more concerned that confidentiality is carefully observed in the day-to-day working environment. It is important that telephone conversations, discussions between staff, or conversations with a patient should not be overheard by other staff, patients or members of the public.

5.2.3   Providers should ensure that the policy guidelines for staff training and practice include precautions to ensure the protection of confidential information (for instance in transfer of confidential information by fax). The provisions of the Data Protection Act must also be included in staff training and operational guidelines.

5.2.4   Older patients should be consulted on their admission to hospital about whom they wish to be informed concerning their medical condition and their progress, and whether a particular person is authorised to speak on the patient's behalf if he/she is no longer able to communicate.

5.3   **PRIVACY AND DIGNITY**

5.3.1   The expectation that the NHS will respect a patient's privacy, dignity, religious and cultural beliefs, at all times and in all places, is stated in the Patient's Charter.

5.3.2   This may be difficult to achieve in practice. There may at times be a conflict between the satisfaction of needs. For instance, in some circumstances the patient may desire more privacy than it is safe to allow.

5.3.3   Respect by staff for privacy and dignity will stem from their attitude towards patients and the culture in which they work. Trusts must have guidelines and procedures for staff to observe (for instance on obtaining the patient's permission for students to be present during their examination or treatment), which reflect the Trust's philosophy of care towards all patients.

5.3.4   Patients should be asked for their preferred form of address[17]. All staff should wear name badges[55] and should introduce themselves and explain what they are going to do. In the case of older people who may have poor eyesight and/or hearing and/or be confused, patience is required from staff. A private room should be available for interviews and discussions with patients and/or carers.

5.4   COMPLAINTS

5.4.1   Extensive publicity has been given to complaints procedures through the Patient's Charter and other publications from the NHS Executive[55],56.

5.4.2   Essential requirements for complaints handling within the NHS are listed in Box 27.

BOX 27

Essential features of complaints handling identified by the NHS Executive[56]:

a. All Trusts, health authorities and primary care practitioners must have an established complaints procedure
b. The procedure must be well publicised
c. The normal time limit for lodging a complaint is within 12 months of the incident, although this is discretionary
d. Trusts and health authorities must have a designated complaints manager
e. Every Trust and health authority must appoint at least one convenor who is a non-executive member of the board
f. The procedure must include a local resolution process
g. The complainant may request an independent review panel following an unsatisfactory outcome of the local resolution process. This must be within 28 days from the report of the local resolution being sent to the complainant

5.4.3   The issue of complaints is dealt with in more detail in the HSA report Focus on Patients[31], which recommends that local complaints procedures should ensure the following features are addressed within all complaints systems.

BOX 28

> **Features of local procedures for complaints, based on the Focus on Patients working group recommendations[31]:**
>
> **a.** Each complaint is dealt with quickly. A prompt reply shows that is taken seriously
> **b.** The complainant is told what is being done
> **c.** The designated officer directly responsible has sufficient authority and status to follow complaints through and ensure that lessons are learnt
> **d.** The complainant is given reasons if the complaint is not upheld
> **e.** The service apologises and accepts the problem if the complaint is upheld
> **f.** Internal action is taken to remedy the situation that led to the complaint
> **g.** Consequent action to improve the service is fed into other relevant service areas
> **h.** Dissemination should also happen where patients or the public have complimented staff on the service provided and where good practice could be replicated

5.4.4   Two aspects of complaints handling are especially important in relation to services for older people.

> **a.** The patient may be too frail or confused to lodge a complaint independently. Staff may therefore be responding to a relative or friend acting on behalf of the patient. In some situations, staff should be prepared to contact a patient advocate (or the local CHC) to assist the patient
> **b.** Complaints, particularly where patients are confused and frightened, or do not have English as their first language, may arise as a result of misunderstandings. Staff working with older people should be aware of any sensory impairments or confusion in the patient that may create difficulties in communication and understanding

5.4.5   The HSA report, Focus on Patients, contains specific standards for responding on behalf of the Trust to complaints. It is particularly important that complainants are kept informed of the progress of any internal inquiry or action arising from their complaint, about what is being done, and the likely timescales for resolution.

5.4.6   There should be local codes of practice, formally agreed between agencies, for complaints handling by staff working on joint service provision.

5.4.7   The formal structure for monitoring all complaints should be linked to a procedure for action to be taken in response to evidence of persistent problems.

5.5   **ETHNIC AND CULTURAL ISSUES**

5.5.1   Although ethnic minorities are mainly concentrated in the inner city areas of the major cities such as London, Birmingham, Bradford, Manchester and Nottingham, ethnic and cultural issues will also require a response in other areas. Persons who settled in the UK during the 1950s and 1960s are now approaching old age. Many have experienced poor living conditions and low incomes throughout their working lives, and face what has been described as a triple jeopardy[57], namely a possibility that they may encounter problems associated with the following:

a. Age

b. Cultural and racial discrimination

c. Lack of access to health, housing and social services

5.5.2 The challenge for the health service stems not simply from the growing numbers of ethnic older persons. Among ethnic groups there is also evidence of a greater prevalence of those health problems associated with poor housing and other issues surrounding social concerns[57].

5.5.3 The response by Social Service departments to the increasing numbers of ethnic older persons has in many cases been an attempt to understand the diversity of cultures they service. In this way issues of race are brought into the mainstream of their considerations[58]. A similar recognition has been made by inner city based NHS services, and this will need to be built upon.

5.5.4 In all contexts a full assessment of the patient's religious and cultural needs is required. The ability of the Trust to meet these needs should be closely monitored in order to establish the level of need locally.

5.5.5 The disease pattern among older persons of ethnic origin does not differ significantly from that of their compatriots. Tropical diseases are relatively rare[57]. Nevertheless the demographic impact of ageing among minority ethnic populations will mean communication and understanding will become increasingly significant issues.

5.5.6 General practitioners may be among practitioners consulted, and will need to be alert to the possibility that alternative medications may be used by the patient. The employment of doctors and practice staff from local ethnic communities is one way to assist an understanding of alternative practices.

5.5.7 There are a number of ways in which the hospital environment can be made more user friendly towards ethnic groups. These are listed in Box 29.

BOX 29

Creating a better hospital environment for patients from different ethnic minority groups[57]:

a. Interpreters available for inpatients and outpatient work

b. Culturally appropriate meals provided

c. Use of directional signs and symbols

d. Booklets, cassette tapes and hospital radio in languages other than English

e. Equal access, information and provision for all patients in discharge planning and follow up

f. Cultural practice relating to death and mourning should be accommodated

g. Equal opportunities policy to address representation of ethnic minorities at all levels of hospital appointments. Minimum requirement of an equal opportunities policy includes the ethnic monitoring of all appointments

5.5.8   It is not possible for staff to be aware of the different needs and requirements of the entire range of ethnic groups. Trusts should draw up a procedure (and provide training in its use) to ensure key issues of importance to patients from ethnic minorities are addressed, and issue this to all staff who have contact with patients. The procedure must set out the questions that should be asked relating to possible treatment (e.g. attitude to pain relief or blood transfusion) diet, form of address, religious beliefs etc.

5.5.9   Staff should be clear about the procedure for accessing the Trust's interpreter service on a 24-hour basis. Where a relative is interpreting, staff should try to confirm that this practice is the patient's preferred option[10].

5.5.10   Use of an information file is recommended on cultural issues that may arise which includes a list of contacts in local communities (e.g. that compiled by Lambeth, Southwark and Lewisham[59]). It should be noted that advance information of cultural needs may assist the prompt provision of services and avoidance of misunderstandings. Significant information should be conveyed along with an initial patient referral.

5.6   ELDER ABUSE

Elder abuse is defined in the DoH document No Longer Afraid (SSI, 1993) as being physical, sexual, psychological or financial. It may be intentional or unintentional or the result of neglect.

Others have drawn attention to the significance of power relationships where the abuse is repeated, and is a violation of a person's human and civil rights by a person or persons who have power over the life of a dependent. Elder abuse may take place in both domestic and institutional settings, and is recognised as a social problem. It may also be racially motivated. Although the main emphasis in Government publications has been on the domestic environment, the possibility of abuse in institutional settings should not be ignored.

5.6.1   All NHS providers must have a policy on elder abuse, with guidance to staff on action to take when elder abuse is suspected of occurring either within an institutional setting or in the domestic environment. It is considered best practice for social services, health services, housing departments and police to jointly prepare and apply a combined strategy to identify and manage elder abuse.

5.6.2   Circumstances within which the incidence of elder abuse may occur, the presence of which should prompt alertness to its possible occurrence, include the following:

    a. Long standing abusive relationships
    b. Patients who suffer from dementia
    c. The older person has a physical illness that affects their mental capacity, continence, mobility
    d. Where there are communication problems due to sensory impairment
    e. Behavioural disturbance
    f. Family stress, for instance due to low income, poor housing, unemployment
    g. History of mental instability, alcohol and/or substance abuse in the care givers

5.6.3 Indications of abuse in the institutional setting could be:

a. Poor standards of hygiene. The older person may be dirty and unkempt and when incontinent smell of urine/faeces
b. Evidence of poor basic personal care e.g. pressure sores, long dirty nails
c. Malnourishment
d. Lack of individual care plans
e. Lack of positive communication from the staff
f. Patronising or bullying attitude of staff towards patients

5.6.4 Health workers in both community and hospital settings should be aware of the warning signs set out above particularly when linked to any of the following presenting conditions in Box 30.

BOX 30

Indicators of elder abuse:

a. The patient displays excessive drowsiness, general unhappiness, flinches or withdraws when approached
b. Bruising/burns to inner arms and thighs, round wrists or ankles
c. Injuries, inconsistent with history given
d. Frequent minor injuries
e. Sexual interference
f. Poor nutrition
g. Prescribed medication not being administered by carer
h. Use of inappropriate medication in order to control behaviour

---

5.6.5 Hospitals are not exempt from the possibility of elder abuse. Factors which may contribute to circumstances wherein abuse within the hospital may occur are given in Box 31 below.

BOX 31

Factors which may lead to abuse within hospital settings include[60]:

a. A poor staff/patient ratio
b. Inappropriate patient mix, e.g. confused patients mixed with those without cognitive impairment
c. Staff not adequately trained to care for patients with physical or mental impairments
d. Inadequate supervision of staff
e. Staff have poor morale
f. Bullying members of staff
g. Ward and staff are isolated within the hospital
h. Frequent use of agency staff

5.6.6 Hospital staff guidance on elder abuse should include advice to staff on action to take if a colleague is suspected of abuse or if abuse is witnessed. A patient or relative/carer who wishes to complain about abuse within the hospital should be encouraged to use the complaints procedure. Other aspects of guidance on elder abuse, which should be readily accessible to staff in the A&E department and on wards, are listed in Box 32.

BOX 32

> **Guidance on action to be taken where elder abuse is suspected should include[61]:**
>
> a. The action to be taken if an older person is believed to be in <u>immediate</u> danger e.g. contacting the police
> b. Recognition of the underlying principle that it is desirable to obtain the patient's consent to any proposed action, although other considerations such as the public interest or possible criminal investigations may also be involved
> c. The recommendation that staff should consult with managers/colleagues as to whether an adult protection referral should be made to social services, or to the Residential Care Homes Inspection Unit/Nursing Homes Registration and Inspection Unit if residential/nursing homes involved
> d. Where a patient reveals that abuse has taken place and asks for help, the manager responsible for reporting to the social services assessment team or Inspection Unit should be immediately informed. A written referral should follow verbal contact within 24 hours

5.6.7   Assessment of the situation should be conducted by a multi-disciplinary team working with social services. Action taken should be with the agreement of the older person, unless they are suffering mental impairment. Once identified, the situation should be monitored by both health and social services. Box 33 lists possible interventions to prevent elder abuse.

BOX 33

> **Possible actions to prevent elder abuse[62]:**
>
> a. Full medical and social assessment to identify possible causes
> b. Respite care
> c. Day care
> d. Home care support
> e. Home adaptations
> f. Nursing support
> g. Continence advice
> h. Family therapy
> i. Rehousing
> j. Referral to the police
> k. Legal advice on protection

Early referral for advocacy, counselling or mediation in situations of internal family conflict or conflict with neighbours may prevent elder abuse happening[63].

Consultation with social services may lead to obtaining legal advice on protection (a series of Acts provide the basis for intervention) or referral to the police. The Department of Health has commissioned national guidelines on the abuse of vulnerable adults which are due to be published in 1999.

5.7   DYING, DEATH AND BEREAVEMENT

5.7.1   Detailed standards for the care of the dying and the clinical care of persons whose condition becomes terminal are contained in separate HSA reports[35],[64]. Two major features of this care are emphasised. First that the care of dying people requires particular care and skill to ensure that their dignity and comfort is preserved. Secondly that the care given to people who are dying must reflect their own choice, which may of course alter with time. The reports contain detailed standards for care of the dying and support to relatives and carers.

5.7.2   Despite the growth of hospice care and terminal care at home, most people die in hospital and 15-20% of older people admitted to acute wards die there. It is therefore important that there should be a hospital wide policy for the care of dying patients[35]. Many hospitals have set up multi-disciplinary terminal care teams[65]. Such a team will offer support and advice on dealing with the terminal symptoms of patients in the hospital. With the agreement of the general practitioner, the team may also provide continuity of care in the home setting.

5.7.3   The following are symptoms that a patient who is dying may experience and which will require immediate assessment and the formulation of a treatment plan within two hours[64].

BOX 34

Symptoms often presented by seriously ill or dying patients:
a. Pain
b. Nausea and vomiting
c. Dyspnoea (difficult or obstructed breathing)
d. Thirst or sore mouth
e. Faecal or urinary incontinence
f. Depression and spiritual distress
g. Constipation
h. Pressure sores and wounds (which may be odorous)
i. Eating difficulties
j. Hiccoughing
k. Fatigue
l. Confusion
m. Communication problems
n. Terminal restlessness

5.7.4   Medical and nursing staff should monitor terminally ill patients on a daily or hourly basis, depending on when death is expected[35].

5.7.5   Specialist advice may be required from the palliative care team, from the clinical pharmacist on medication, from the dietician and/or speech and language therapist for resolving eating difficulties, and from a counsellor or chaplain for treating depression and giving spiritual advice.

5.7.6   The patient's relatives (or carer) should be able to speak to the doctor soon after admission, so that they can be made aware of the prognosis for the patient. Giving such information requires the patient's consent.

5.7.7   The decision of the doctor on whether to attempt resuscitation should be taken in consultation with the patient (if competent and willing) and with relatives/carers/nursing staff, and be recorded in the patient's notes. Where known the patient's wishes should be taken into account and in particular the existence and terms of a living will[66] (see also 3.4.2). Trust policy on resuscitation must not automatically exclude resuscitation on the grounds of age.

5.7.8   Dying patients should be allowed 24-hour visiting facilities for a relative or carer to sit with them through the night if the patient wishes. Sleeping accommodation and access to meals should be available.

5.7.9   Relatives, particularly in the case of older people, may have been caring for the patient for some time. Staff should encourage their continued involvement with the day to day practical care of the patient.

5.7.10   The patient has the right to discharge him/herself. Thus wherever possible the hospital staff should support the wish of the dying patient to go home, providing the responsible clinician is satisfied with the level of support the patient will receive, and provided the relatives/carers agree. In particular continuity of care must be maintained.

5.7.11   The general practitioner must be informed within 24 hours of the admission of a terminally ill patient to hospital, and immediately informed if the patient is discharged home or has died in hospital.

5.7.12   The general practitioner is responsible for ensuring that the necessary support services are available to the dying patient who is at home. The level of support may vary but there should be access to 24-hour nursing support.

5.7.13   Inevitably the likelihood of losing close relatives and friends increases with age. The grief felt by the death of a life long partner or friend may seem insurmountable to the bereaved person. Many hospitals provide practical advice to the bereaved on registering the death and arranging the funeral. Where the surviving partner is him/herself confused and/or in poor health, hospital staff should ensure that practical assistance, either from friends or a voluntary agency, is available. All hospitals should provide copies of the DSS booklet What to do after a death in England and Wales or What to do after a death in Scotland or, Practical advice for time of bereavement (also in Scotland).

5.7.14   There should be a Trust wide procedure for hospital staff that covers viewing the body, collection of possessions and obtaining the death certificate.

5.7.15   Staff who have been involved in caring for the patient should make themselves available, by appointment, to discuss any issues with the bereaved.

6 Strategies for responding to the issue of falls

Falls occur both within the community, whether at home or in institutional environments (care homes or nursing homes), and within acute care facilities. This section on strategies for the avoidance of falls among the elderly addresses the issue within both environments, looking first at methods of preventing falls in the community and identifying the role of the primary health care team (6.1) and then presenting a strategy for avoiding the occurrence of falls in hospital (6.2) taken from the HSA report on Emergency Medical Admissions (section 3.1.3).

6.1 A STRATEGY FOR PREVENTING FALLS IN THE COMMUNITY SETTING

Falls are a serious public health problem among older people. 30% of people over 65 years of age fall each year[67]. Unintentional injury, most often caused by a fall, is the sixth leading cause of death among people over 65 years of age. The incidence of falls rises with age. Falling is twice as common among women. A multifactorial strategy of risk factor abatement has recently been shown to reduce the risk of falling. Some falls are pure accidents but repeated falling should be taken as a warning of poor health status and investigated accordingly.

6.1.1 A number of studies have been undertaken on the prevention of falls. These have focused on three areas:

a. Exercise particularly balancing, low impact aerobics and muscle strengthening
b. Home visiting, to advise on reducing the risk of falling in the home. This may be undertaken by health visitors, nurses, occupational therapists and physiotherapists. This could include referral for local authority funding for minor improvements in the home to make it safer (see also 2.15.9)
c. Diet, in particular the introduction of high dose vitamin D supplements and calcium equivalent to half a pint of milk a day reduce the risk of fracture

6.1.2 The risk of falling increases with age. Those living alone, with continence problems or on drugs with side effects, may have an increased risk of falling. Health checks by general practitioners for those over 75 years of age should include assessment of this risk. Other aspects of a falls prevention programme would include health visiting to identify risk in the home environment, and work with occupational therapists and physiotherapists on reducing identified risk factors.

6.1.3 The following are indicators which should be addressed when screening patients for comprehensive assessment of their risk of falling and the development of an individually tailored falls prevention plan (see also 3.4.7 above and 6.1..5 below).

a. The patient lives alone
b. The spouse/partner is unable to provide support
c. The patient has a dementia syndrome
d. Patients with Parkinson's Disease or syndrome
e. A cerebrovascular accident has occurred
f. The patient has a walking impairment
g. The patient has cardiovascular disease
h. The patient has arthritis/cervical spondylosis
i. The patient may be making excessive use of sedatives, tranquillisers, diuretics etc.
j. The patient has a continence problem

6.1.4   Comprehensive assessment must include a full medical assessment of each patient who presents with unexplained or repeated falls or who presents with one or more of the risk indicators listed above (6.1.3).

  a. All patients need a full medical assessment to identify any specific treatable causes of falling, and a multi-disciplinary assessment once these have been excluded
  b. Patients without obvious treatable medical causes for falls require occupational therapy and/or physiotherapy assessment for risk factors
  c. If visual or hearing impairments are detected, further assessment of the impairment is required.

6.1.5   The following management pathway should be adopted and implemented by primary health care teams, as soon as investigation/medical intervention has either excluded or resolved any clinical causes of falling.

  a. Assessment of visual acuity and hearing (this may be performed by a specialist nurse or by a community optician/audiologist)
  b. Assessment of mobility, balance and gait within the home by a physiotherapist/health visitor/occupational therapist/nurse
  c. Assessment of appropriate footwear or foot problems
  d. Occupational therapy assessment - safety of transfers to bath/toilet, environmental hazards e.g. furniture (incorrect height, unstable)
  e. Review of medication and compliance once home. This may include advice from pharmacist on side effects of medication
  f. Assessment of family and social circumstances and needs for social care
  g. Rehabilitation of muscle strength and balance through exercise
  h. Need for some form of community alarm
  i. Installation of structures e.g. grab bars or handrails
  j. Review of diet perhaps leading to dietary/vitamin supplements to reduce risk of fractures

6.2   A STRATEGY FOR AVOIDING FALLS IN HOSPITAL SETTINGS

Avoidable patient falls impact on medical management, delay discharge, lead to complications and additional treatment, increase the risk of litigation, increase post-discharge dependency with higher risk of ensuing re-admission and above all cause unnecessary patient suffering. Studies of the causes, effects and costs of patient falls[67] lead the working group to recommend the adoption of specific falls avoidance strategies.

To ensure care is provided in a safe environment the following procedures should be adopted.

6.2.1   Trusts should work to a falls prevention policy which requires the collection of data on all patient falls. This data should be used to generate regular information on falls analysed by patient age, medical condition, location, time of fall and related circumstances such as continence problems, wandering, or the effects of medication.

6.2.2   Each Trust's training and education programmes for medical and nursing staff should include reference to the falls issue; the assessment of a patient's risk of falling and measures to prevent avoidable falls.

6.2.3   All patients should be assessed to determine their risk of falling. Recognising the link between falls and incontinence and between incontinence and tissue viability, the working group recommends the advantages of composite patient assessment regarding continence, tissue viability and the risk of falling being conducted with all patients on admission.

Following assessment, patients identified as being of high risk of falling should benefit from targeted care focusing on their risk factors. Such care must not compromise their privacy, personal dignity or right to give or withhold consent to treatments.

6.2.4   The risk management programmes applied in all Trusts should include periodic reviews from the falls prevention perspective, identifying potential risk factors in the care environment or within clinical or support procedures. Systems should be in place to ensure note is taken of identified risks and appropriate action taken.

6.2.5   All Trusts should have written guidelines setting out practice and procedures to reduce risks of falls in all care areas. There should be written guidelines for specific targeted care for high risk patients, and care plans focusing on risk of falling should be part of such patients' notes. Patients', carers' and visitors' understanding and co-operation regarding falls prevention can be supported by falls avoidance leaflets, posters etc.

6.2.6   Trusts should explore available technologies to support staff caring for high risk patients. Spontaneous call systems or movement monitors should be considered.

7 Strategies for the care of older patients with a dementia syndrome

Dementia is the common term used for a group of diseases that affect the normal working functions of the brain... characterised by a decline in intellectual, physical and memory functions, along with changes in personality and a deterioration in social functioning[68]. It is always of long duration, usually progressive and irreversible. It occurs predominantly within the elderly population[69].

Dementia presents in a continuum of severity[70] and the following categories give a rough indication of the varying levels of support required.

Mild - work and social activity is significantly limited but the capacity for independent living is retained.

Moderate - independent living is hazardous and some degree of supervision is needed.

Severe - continual supervision is needed and the patient cannot maintain minimal personal hygiene.

It is also important to note that the patient may retain the capacity for decision-making for some time after the initial diagnosis. Patients who receive a diagnosis in the early stages should discuss with their doctor the information which may be given to family and carers, in order to protect their right to confidentiality. Mild dementia may not be incompatible with the ability to give informed consent[71]. Approximately 10% of patients over 75 years old suffer from dementia and the proportion increases to around 20% among those over 85.

Patients with a dementia syndrome may as a result encounter problems in the course of maintaining independent or dependent living within the community or in nursing or care home environments. Their difficulties may be compounded when they have health needs requiring on-going management/treatment in the community. Strategies for diagnosing and responding to a dementia syndrome in the community context, both as the principal presenting need, and as a factor within any combination of co-existing illnesses, are set out in section 7.1. A strategy for acute services to ensure the quality of care they provide to older patients with dementia, is set out in section 7.2 (largely taken from HSA's report on Emergency Medical Admissions (section 10.4))[35].

7.1 MANAGING DEMENTIA IN THE COMMUNITY

Under the NHS and Community Care Act 1990 Social Service departments are required to invite health and housing authorities to assist in the assessment of needs. Diagnosis of dementia, however, will generally be made by a consultant in the psychiatry of old age, a consultant geriatrician or sometimes by a consultant neurologist. There is, therefore, a requirement from the early stages for close co-operation between the secondary and primary health care sectors and with social services, if the patient and carer is to receive the appropriate level of support, and to access the relevant services when they are needed.

7.1.1 Early diagnosis is important in order to plan appropriate support for the patient and carer as well as to provide the opportunity for therapeutic intervention. A number of measures can be taken to facilitate the identification of cases, such as[68]:

a. Providing information to the public about dementia and how to access appropriate services

b. Agreement between health and social services on who should manage the standardised assessment of persons believed to have a dementia syndrome

c. The selection of 'trigger' questions to be raised during community care assessments which may identify the presence of dementia

d. Clear referral route to secondary specialist care

e. A preliminary diagnosis of dementia may be made with a recognised test of cognitive function and a medical check by the general practitioner

f. Screening of over 75 year olds for dementia

7.1.2   The objectives of health care for patients with dementia should be to:

a. Identify and treat reversible causes of cognitive impairment

b. Provide an early diagnosis to allow the introduction of possible new therapies

c. Reduce the carer's burdens and stress

d. Reduce the psychological distress of the patient

e. Arrange access to support services

f. Co-operate with other support agencies

7.1.3   NHS services which should be available to patients with a diagnosed dementia syndrome and to their carers, include:

a. A needs assessment, including a discussion of the diagnosis and prognosis with the patient and carer

b. The treatment of co-existing illnesses

c. Information and advice about treatment, medication and support services available

d. Community support such as monitoring by the community psychiatric nurse, day hospital services at need and respite care

e. Memory clinics (provided in some areas)

7.1.4   Informal carers have a central role in the daily life of patients with dementia and the provision of support on health related issues and access to respite care are important elements of a sustained programme of care[72].

7.2   **CARING FOR PATIENTS WITH DEMENTIA IN THE ACUTE SECTOR**

It is important to ensure that the admission of patients known to be suffering from a dementia syndrome is appropriately managed in three critical areas, namely the process of admission through A&E or an admissions ward on to the appropriate general medical ward or special care unit (7.2.1); the adoption and implementation of evidence based guidelines (7.2.2); the crucially important area of communications with patients and their relatives and carers (7.2.3).

7.2.1   Admission through A&E or an admissions ward can be a particularly confusing and distressing experience for patients with a dementia syndrome and best practice will provide a quiet room for initial assessment and the taking of admitting notes, if appropriate. A full social history, including support arrangements, must be documented on admission. This is greatly facilitated by the presence of a relative or carer. Admitting notes taken must include information on the patient's previous cognitive state, the findings of a mental state examination (the abbreviated mental test score) and notes on the patient's previous level of function. General practitioners referring patients for admission must ensure they provide as much of this relevant information as is available to them at the time of referral. Where patients present independently at the hospital the medical admitting team is responsible for gathering all relevant information from whatever sources are available and for contacting the patient's general practitioner to inform them of their patient's admission and to obtain any information otherwise unavailable to them. Contact with the general practitioner will take place during the working day (9 a.m. - 5 p.m.).

7.2.2   The Trust should produce and apply joint clinical guidelines for the admission and management of patients with dementia. These guidelines should include reference to medical assessment, social history, the selection and conduct of an appropriate and authoritative mental state assessment questionnaire and the indications for referral to a consultant psychiatrist (drawn up by the liaison psychiatrist). The management of patients with dementia should feature in the educational programme for doctors in training.

These joint guidelines must incorporate an arrangement to ensure the patient's urgent access to the liaison psychiatry team where this is appropriate. There must also be a procedure whereby the admitting team may refer patients with dementia to social services and also to the community psychiatric nursing service. Social services or the community psychiatric nursing service will be expected to begin their assessments of the patient on the day of admission or the next day (unless it is clinically inappropriate to do so).

7.2.3   Communicating information, instructions and advice, and consulting with patients and their relatives and carers, requires particularly robust attention in the case of patients suffering from a dementia syndrome. Mechanisms should be in place which support verbal with written information, and the giving of information must be recorded in the notes. Patients, relatives or carers must be fully consulted on the drawing up of care plans and advised/trained to participate in their delivery as appropriate. Social services and mental health services will have their own local policies to meet the care programme approach to post-discharge care. Discharge procedures developed to provide for patients with dementia should accommodate a local understanding of the implications of these policies.

8 Management of stroke

The high incidence and serious consequences of stroke make it one of the most important challenges faced by contemporary medicine. In the UK stroke is one of the three main causes of death, and a major cause of long-term disability. As a result it consumes more NHS resources than any other condition.

This statement on the significance of stroke and its impact on patients and their families comes from the Royal College of Physicians of Edinburgh Consensus Statement, 1998.

What follows addresses the management of stroke from the particular perspective of the older patient, draws on the HSA report Service Standards for Emergency Medical Admissions, 1997[35]; The Royal College of Physicians of Edinburgh Consensus Statement and the Clinical Standards Advisory Group (CSAG) report, 1998[73].

8.1 CORE STANDARDS FOR THE MANAGEMENT OF STROKE

The following key standards address the prime features of the management of stroke and should be adopted and met by all Trusts seeking to ensure they deliver the best quality of care to their stroke patients.

8.1.1 Care of patients with acute stroke must be on the main site of the acute general hospital, preferably in a specialist unit for acute care and rehabilitation.

8.1.2 Supervision must be provided by a consultant physician or geriatrician with a special interest in stroke and with easy access to specialist advice in cardiology and neurology. Cover must be provided during this co-ordinating consultant's absence. Many of the skills required for the best management of stroke patients are among those possessed by geriatricians.

8.1.3 The consultant should co-ordinate a multi-disciplinary team which includes specialist nursing, a speech and language therapist, an occupational therapist and a physiotherapist specialising in neurology. The team needs to have formally arranged access to clinical psychology, continence advice, counselling and social services. Meetings of the team should be held at least weekly to co-ordinate patient care. The team's function is to provide for the patient's assessment, treatment, care and discharge planning.

8.1.4 The team should use agreed protocols covering the assessment and management of stroke patients, which specify the investigations required, set out the indications for investigation and treatment, and include the methods of clinical management to be adopted by the team.

8.1.5 The investigation and management of acute stroke should be in accordance with evidence based clinical guidelines (e.g. Scottish Intercollegiate Guidelines Network (SIGN)). The Clinical Standards Advisory Group and Royal College of Physicians of Edinburgh reports already referred to, provide useful guidance.

8.1.6 The supplementary clinical services which must be available to support the work of the multi-disciplinary stroke team described in 8.1.3 above are detailed in Box 35. Access to these services should be set out in written agreements between them and the stroke team, including reference to availability and response to referral timescales.

BOX 35

Clinical support services in collaboration with the stroke team include:

a. Access to specialist nursing advice for specific problems, e.g. continence, prevention of pressure sores
b. Provision of therapy services (including clinical psychology, dietetics, occupational therapy, physiotherapy, speech and language therapy) consistent with professional guidance
c. A designated social worker/care manager attached to the stroke team or other arranged social work support

---

8.1.7 All Trusts admitting patients with stroke must ensure that members of the stroke team, both nursing and medical, receive continuing professional education/training. In-house training on the management of stroke must be given to all clinical staff whose duties include care for stroke patients.

8.1.8 Protocols/guidelines adopted for the management of stroke (see 8.1.5 above) must contain reference to the key features set out in Box 36 below:

BOX 36

Management of stroke patients in hospital:

a. Each patient must have a full, recorded, neurological assessment on admission using an agreed protocol
b. An urgent brain scan is indicated within 24 hours if:
   i)   a cerebellar or subarachnoid haemorrhage is suspected
   ii) the patient is on anti-coagulation therapy
   iii) thrombolytic or anti-coagulation therapy is being considered
c. A CT brain scan should be conducted whenever the findings might influence management, particularly to resolve doubts as to whether the event is ischaemic or haemorrhagic
d. Antiplatelet therapy, normally aspirin, must be prescribed immediately for patients who have ischaemic stroke
e. Routine screening within 24 hours with a standardised screening procedure (swallow test) to check for dysphagia
f. Hydration and nutrition needs must be routinely assessed
g. Agreed standardised measures to assess functional ability (including pre-morbid function and post-stroke disability)
h. Continence must be assessed and patterns of incontinence monitored
i. Formal recording of the patient's mood must be undertaken
j. Routine screening with a standardised procedure to check for cognitive deficits, i.e. perception, concentration and memory
k. External compression stockings should be used for the prevention of deep vein thrombosis in stroke patients with impaired mobility

---

8.1.9   Communication between clinical staff and their patients and their patients' carers is crucial. The expertise of the speech and language therapist may be required to ensure that the patient can communicate effectively. Particular care is required in presenting choices/options for treatment and care. Individualised goals should be drawn up, checked and agreed with patients/carers.

Information on stroke diagnosis and treatment, secondary prevention, services for stroke rehabilitation and welfare rights and financial benefits should be readily available and given to patients/carers verbally and in written form.

The stroke unit or Trust should have established links with patient/carer interest groups, particularly those specialising in stroke, with arrangements in place whereby these services can be accessed by patients and/or their carers.

8.1.10   Discharge planning and care must be in accordance with the standards set out in HSA's report Service Standards for Discharge Care[6] supplemented with standards set out in this report on the care of older people. In particular:

a. Patients and carers must be involved at an early stage and discharge arrangements should be agreed with the patient and/or carer
b. The need for help at home and training for carers in the use of equipment (if discharge to home is envisaged as a medium or longer term goal), must be identified with the patient and/or carer at an early stage. Referrals to occupational therapy for home adaptations and equipment and to case managers for home care packages should also be made at the earliest opportunity
c. Information given to the patient must include:
    i)   A named contact to whom the patient may refer after discharge. (This may be a key worker in the hospital unit, a discharge liaison worker, social worker or member of the primary health care team)
    ii) The patient's own written discharge summary
    iii) A written post-discharge care plan
    iv) Information regarding resources in the community, including information on statutory and voluntary agencies
    v)   Information about who will contact them after discharge, and when (e.g. within 48 hours, one week, one month etc.), to follow up on the patient's progress
d. By the day of discharge the general practitioner is informed of the patient's diagnosis, medication, plans for future care and management and community services arranged
e. If the patient is not able to be discharged home, standard procedures for arranging continuing care must be followed

8.1.11   There should be agreed protocols with local general practitioners and social services on the follow up of stroke patients, which set out:

a. How patients are to be medically managed following discharge
b. Specified intervals for follow up review appointments at the hospital
c. Community support in the home
d. Rehabilitation services available to patients in the community

8.1.12   All hospitals admitting stroke patients should participate in an established, evidence-based clinical audit scheme such as that developed by the Royal College of Physicians of London for the purposes of monitoring and benchmarking the quality of their service[74].

Procedures should be in place within the Trust to audit the incidence of pressure sores, and to detect hospital acquired chest infections and urinary tract infections in patients with acute stroke, as well as to monitor the number of patients admitted for stroke, their length of stay, numbers discharged and their destinations at discharge.

9 Assuring the quality of the service

The standards contained in this volume represent valid markers of safe and effective care for older people and provide a basis on which providers of such services can develop their clinical governance strategy in this area of care. The complementary accreditation instrument, when published, will provide a practical work book for the implementation of these standards within a structured framework; a framework which establishes a perspective on the initial quality of service, maps out strategies and procedures for improvement, and offers a tool for verifying achievement. Within this framework clinical audit and the monitoring of service delivery play a key role.

All service providers should conduct regular, systematic and multi-professional clinical audit of the care they provide. Their audit programmes should be built around a core of essential topics which address the prime features of their service from the perspectives of clinical risk, the volume of the incidence of presenting conditions, or the significant consumption of resources. Audits should be conducted according to sound methods and their findings clearly presented. Audit programmes should include regular opportunities for the discussion and review of audits undertaken, leading where indicated to action to remedy any weaknesses in care provision identified. The National Centre for Clinical Audit (NCCA) offers advice and assistance on the implementation of a clinical audit programme.

9.1 AUDIT ISSUES IN BOTH COMMUNITY AND ACUTE SECTORS

9.1.1 Routine audit and monitoring by all providers of services to older people must address patients' complaints and comments; the implementation of policies on health and safety; accident reporting and investigation; COSHH practice and waste disposal procedures; infection control policy and practice; the take-up of staff training and continuing education, and overall adherence to the provider's policies and procedures, in particular those covering screening and assessments determining patient eligibility for continuing care.

9.1.2 Particular areas which providers of services to older people are advised to include in their core clinical audit programmes will vary depending on whether the provider functions within the community or is an acute sector service.

9.2 CLINICAL AUDIT AND SERVICE MONITORING IN THE ACUTE SECTOR

9.2.1 Departments of geriatric medicine should ensure that their Trust's audit programme includes audit of the time taken from a decision to admit a patient in A&E to that patient's reaching the ward.

9.2.2 Departments should also ensure their Trust monitors the appropriate referral to (and uptake of) investigations and treatments of older people especially those aged over 75, to determine whether older people enjoy equity of access to care.

9.2.3 Departments should also ensure that the movement or 'out-posting' of older people between wards and their transfer between different clinical teams is subject to systematic tracking, and that both the effectiveness of these systems and the incidence of patient movement is audited.

9.2.4 In the area of clinical management departments should audit patient access to gastroenterological investigation and percutaneous endoscopic gastronomy and in particular audit the insertion of gastronomy tubes.

9.2.5   Other key audits to be undertaken include the Royal College of Physicians clinical audit of stroke management[74]; the incidence of pressure sores; the incidence of hospital acquired chest and urinary tract infections; and the numbers of patients admitted for stroke, their length of stay, and numbers discharged (and to where).

9.3   **CLINICAL AUDIT AND SERVICE MONITORING IN THE COMMUNITY**

9.3.1   Key topics for attention within clinical audit programmes addressing the care of older people within the community include the monitoring of uptake of health promotion and accident prevention services; monitoring the conduct of risk assessments into the likelihood of falls and other accidents by older people at home; the rehabilitation of patients after falls; and the audit of the quality of discharge care planning and practice, post inpatient or day hospital management.

9.3.2   Community sector audit programmes should address compliance with drug and therapeutic regimes by older patients; prescribing patterns and practice for the elderly; and the management of repeat and multiple prescribing.

Appendix I - Membership of the Older People Service Standards Working Group

Dr Gillian Dalley (Chair)
Director
Centre for Policy on Ageing

Ms Sarah Andrews
Co-Director of Nursing
Camden and Islington Community Health
Services Trust

Mr John Bradshaw
Senior Administrator
Lambeth Healthcare NHS Trust

Dr Stuart Bruce
Consultant Physician
Hastings and Rother NHS Trust

Ms Mary Burkett
Associate Director
Lambeth, Southwark and Lewisham Health
Authority

Dr Chris Drinkwater
Senior Lecturer in Primary Health Care
University of Newcastle

Ms Margaret Edwards
Department Planning Manager
London Borough of Richmond upon Thames

Ms Cathinka Guldberg
Chief Speech and Language Therapist
Optimum Health Services Trust

Dr David Goss
General Practitioner (retired)
Welwyn Garden City

Ms Pat Graham
Senior Nurse in Medicine
University Hospital Lewisham

Ms Sarah Hadley
Standards Development and Research Officer
Health Services Accreditation

Mr P Hamlin
Senior Dental Officer
Specialising in Gerodontics
Hailsham Health Centre

Mrs Ann Hare
Senior Nurse, Professional Policy & Practice
Eastbourne Hospitals NHS Trust

Dr Ian Hastie
Senior Lecturer and Consultant Physician
Department of Geriatric Medicine
St George's Medical School

Ms Peggy Hoskins
Senior Physiotherapist
Frimley Park Hospitals NHS Trust

Ms Christine Hughes
South Kent Community Health Council

Ms Suzy Jacob
Service Manager, Elderly Services
Enfield Community Care NHS Trust

Mr Tony Jenkins
Director of Standards Development
Health Services Accreditation

Reverend Hillary Johnson
Chaplain's Office
St. George's Healthcare NHS Trust

Dr Roger Lewis
Consultant in Medicine for the Elderly
Guy's & St. Thomas' Hospital NHS Trust

Dr Brendan O'Connor
Consultant in Public Health Medicine
East Sussex, Brighton and Hove Health
Authority

Dr Sudhir Patel
General Practitioner
Gillingham

Dr Allyson Pollock
Consultant in Public Health Medicine
Merton, Sutton & Wandsworth Health Authority

Dr Fiona Ramsey
Consultant Physician
The Surrey & Sussex Healthcare NHS Trust

Mrs Christine Smith
Professional Supervisor for District Nursing
Optimum Health Services Trust

Ms Kate Squance
Dietician
Guy's and St Thomas's NHS Trust

Dr Ian Starke
Consultant Physician and Senior Lecturer
University Hospital Lewisham

Ms Barbara Stranc
Commissioning Manager
Merton, Sutton and Wandsworth Health
Authority

Mr Brendan Ward
Acting Director of Strategic &
Service Development
NHS Executive - South Thames RHA

Ms Margaret Whittington
Service Manager
Bromley Social Services

Mrs Angela Wilson
Director of Clinical and Therapy Services
East Kent Community NHS Trust

Mrs Frances Winterborn
Former Manager
Battle Carers

Dr Ginny Wright
Consultant Physician
Richmond, Twickenham & Roehampton
Healthcare NHS Trust

**Community based services group
- additional membership**

Ms J Robinson
Adult Community Physiotherapist
North Downs Community Health NHS Trust

Dr E Aitken
Consultant Physician
University Hospital, Lewisham

*Members of the working groups attended and
participated in a personal and individual capacity.*

Appendix II - Contributors to the consultative process

Mr Greg Applegate
Assistant Director, Acute Commissioning
Croydon Health Authority

Mrs E M Bamford
Head of Adult Provider Services
Social Services - West Sussex County Council

Dr Bannerjee
Policy and Executive committee member
British Geriatrics Society

Dr David Black
Consultant Geriatrician
Chairman College Committee on Geriatrics
Queen Mary's Sidcup NHS Trust

Ms Sue Botes
Professional Officer
Community Practitioners' & Health Visitors'
Association

Ms Joanna Brown
Director of Industrial Relations & Professional
Practice
The Society of Chiropodists and Podiatrists

Ms Karen Bryan
Royal College of Speech and Language
Therapists

Ms Angeline Burke
Development Officer
Association of Community Health Councils for
England & Wales

Dr G R Burston
Chair Bristol and District CHC
Bristol & District Community Health Council

Dr Tim Carter
Medical Adviser, Primary Care Development
West Sussex Health Authority

Mr Steve Cody
Assistant Director, Adult Services Division
Social Services, London Borough of Lambeth

Dr J A Coles
Consultant Physician
St George's Healthcare NHS Trust

Ms Gill Collinson
Assistant Regional Nurse Director
NHS Executive - Anglia & Oxford

Mrs Yvonne Craig
London

Mrs A M Dean
Chief Executive
Dartford & Gravesham NHS Trust

Mr J E Deft
Joint Chief Officer
Lancaster and Morecambe Community Health
Council

Dr Edward Dickinson
Director (Acting)
Royal College of Physicians of London

Dr John Duffy
Consultant Physician Medicine & Elderly Care
Winchester & Eastleigh Healthcare NHS Trust

Mr Mervyn Eastman
Director of Social Services & Member of ADDSS
Older People's Committee
London Borough of Enfield Social Services

Ms A Edwards
District Nurse
St Leonards-on-Sea, East Sussex

Ms Pam Evans
Royal College of Speech & Language Therapists

Ms Lesley Forester
Locality Director Guildford
Surrey Hampshire Borders NHS Trust

Ms Sue Gallagher
Chief Executive
Merton, Sutton and Wandsworth Health
Authority

Mr Peter Gilroy
Strategic Director of Social Services
Kent County Council

Mrs E Gladman
Assistant Director of Nursing
Hastings & Rother NHS Trust

Mr Roger M Goss
'Patientline' Manager
The Patients Association

Mr Tony Griffiths
Director of Care Community & Older People
Services
Merton & Sutton Community NHS Trust

Mr D Heller
Project Manager
Ashford St Peter's Hospitals NHS Trust

Dr Hendra
Policy and Executive committee member
British Geriatrics Society

Ms Elizabeth Housden
Secretary, General Practitioners Committee
British Medical Association

Dr Warwick Hunt
Medical Adviser
Northamptonshire Health Authority

Ms Glennis Jaques
Clinical Nurse Manager
Acute & Elderly Medicine
Northern General Hospital NHS Trust

Ms Debra Jeffery
Secretary to the Chief Medical Officer
Department of Health

Ms Soline Jerram
Nurse Practitioner
Chichester Priority Care Services NHS Trust

Dr Kafetz
Policy and Executive committee member
British Geriatrics Society

Dr Kennie
Policy and Executive committee member
British Geriatrics Society

Mrs Lesley Knight
Health Visitor for Older People
Worcestershire Community Healthcare
NHS Trust

Ms Julie Lowe
Service Director: Medicine
Greenwich Healthcare NHS Trust

Mr M J Lowe
Deputy Secretary
British Medical Association

Dr D G MacMahon (and colleagues)
Consultant Physician
Chair, British Geriatrics Society Policy
Committee

Mr Brendan McCormack
Head of Practice Development & Co-Director,
Gerontological Nursing Programme
Royal College of Nursing

Dr Elizabeth McInnes
Consultant Physician in Care of the Elderly
Ashford St Peter's Hospitals NHS Trust

Councillor Gill Mitchell
Brighton & Hove

Mr I W Nixon
Planning Manager
Kingston & Richmond Health Authority

Ms Jean O'Shaughnessy
Chief Officer
Mid Surrey Community Health Council

Ms Gwyneth Owen
Professional Adviser
The Chartered Society of Physiotherapy

Ms Jean Pearson
Dietetic Services Manager
Nottingham Community Health NHS Trust

Dr Bill Reith
Honorary Secretary of Council
Royal College of General Practitioners

Miss L A Roberts
Consultant in Accident & Emergency
Kent & Sussex Weald NHS Trust

Mr L A Ruben
South Thames East, Department of Postgraduate
General Practice Education

Mr M L Savage
Director of Accreditation
Health Services Accreditation

Dr Theo Schofield
Division of Public Health & Primary Care
Oxford University - Institute of Health Sciences

Mr Anthony P Smith
Chief Executive
English National Board for Nursing, Midwifery
& Health Visiting

Dr David G Smithard
Consultant in Elderly and Stroke Medicine,
South Kent Hospitals NHS Trust

Ms Sheelah Soopramania (and colleagues)
Service Leader-Elderly (MH)
Surrey Oaklands NHS Trust

Mrs S J Stevens
Head of Speech & Language Therapy
The Hammersmith Hospitals NHS Trust

Ms Jenny Stiles
Director
The Relatives Association

Ms Melanie Summers
General Manager Medicine
Geriatric Medicine & Cardiothoracic Services
St George's Healthcare NHS Trust

Dr J St J Thomas
Fellow and Secretary
Royal College of Physicians of Edinburgh

Dr Jan Wagstyl
St James's Practice
Beckenham, Kent

Dr S Watkins
Senior Medical Officer
Welsh Office

Dr Linda Watt
Medical Director
Greater Glasgow Community & Mental Health
Services NHS Trust

Dr Jane Wilkinson
Senior Medical Officer
Welsh Office

Ms Colleen Williams
Joint Commissioning Manager
West Surrey Health Authority

HSA gratefully acknowledges the additional help and assistance received from the following:

Mrs Belinda Banham CBE
London

Ginny Jenkins
Action on Elder Abuse

Jean Pearson
Nottingham Community Health NHS Trust

Mrs S J Stevens
Hammersmith Hospitals NHS Trust

The Health Education Authority

Appendix III - References

1. The Audit Commission. The Coming of Age. London: 1997.

2. Department of Health. A First Class Service: Quality in the New NHS. London: DoH, 1998.

3. SSI/Department of Health. Better Management, Better Care. Sixth Annual Report of the Chief Inspector Social Services Inspectorate. London: HMSO, 1996/97.

4. EL(96)8. NHS Responsibilities for meeting continuing health care needs - current progress and future priorities. 1996.

5. Health Services Accreditation. Standards for Accident and Emergency Services (third edition). Battle: HSA, 1996.

6. Health Services Accreditation. Standards for Discharge Care. Battle: HSA, 1996.

7. HSG(95)8. NHS Responsibilities for Meeting Continuing Health Care Needs. 1995.

8. NHSE. The New NHS Modern Dependable. CM3807. HMSO, December 1997.

9. Health Services Accreditation. Standards for Continence Services. Battle: HSA, 1997.

10. The British Medical Association/The Royal College of Nursing. The Older Person: Consent and Care. London: BMA, 1995.

11. NHS and Community Care Act. London: HMSO, 1990.

12. NICE work for GPs? General Practitioner. 6 November 1998: 1.

13. Pushpangadan M, Burns E. Caring for Older People. Community Services: Health. British Medical Journal. 1996.

14. AGILE, ACPC, OCTEP. Guidelines for the Collaborative Rehabilitation Management of Elderly People Who Have Fallen.

15. Health Services Accreditation. Standards for primary care services: Pharmaceutical services in the community. Battle: HSA, (in preparation January 1999).

16. Health Services Accreditation. Standards for NHS Pharmacy in Hospital and Community Health Services. Battle: 1998.

17. Department of Health. The Patient's Charter. London: HMSO, 1991 (revised 1995).

18. Standards of Medical Care for Older People: Expectations and Recommendations. BGS Compendium, Document D3 (1995).

19. Department of Health. Partnership in Action. A Discussion Document. 1998.

20. EL(97)62. Better Services for Vulnerable People.

21. Standardised Assessment Scales for Elderly People. RCP/BGS. 1992.

22. Higginson I, Victor C. Assessment and Screening of Older People. Royal Society of Medicine. 1994.

23. Good Practice Identified by Research: Users Needs and Circumstances. Care Plan. 1996; March.

24. The Royal College of Physicians. Geriatric Day Hospitals. 1994.

25. House of Commons. Health Committee. Third Report. Long-Term Care: Future Provision and Funding. Vol.1. HMSO, July 1996.

26. Caldecourt F. Risk in the Community. Managing Risk. 1993; January.

27. NHS Management Executive. Risk Management in the NHS. London: DoH, 1993.

28. The United Kingdom Central Council for Nursing, Midwifery and Health Visiting. Issues Arising from Professional Conduct Complaints. UKCC 1996; November.

29. Irvine S, Harman H. Making Sense of Personnel Management. Radcliffe Medical Press 1997.

30. Health Services Accreditation. Standards for Outpatient Services. Battle: HSA, 1997.

31. Health Services Accreditation. Focus on Patients: Standards to improve the patient's experience. Battle: HSA, 1998.

32. Health Services Accreditation. Standards for Patient Transport Services. Battle: HSA, 1998.

33. Department of Health. Our Healthier Nation. 1998.

34. HEA. Preventing Home Accidents among Older People. A summary of the process findings and outcomes of a six month exploratory study. HEA 1998.

35. Health Services Accreditation. Standards for Emergency Medical Admissions. Battle: HSA, 1997.

36. Stuck AE, Siu AL, Wieland GD, Adams J, Rubenstein LZ. Comprehensive geriatric assessment: a meta-analysis of controlled trials. Lancet 1993; 342: 1032-6.

37. Rockwood K, Silvius JL, Fox RA. Comprehensive geriatric assessment. Postgraduate Medicine 1998; 103: 247-64.

38. Ferrell BR, Ferrell BA. eds. Pain in the Elderly. International Association for the Study of Pain. IASP Press, 1996.

39. Standards of Medical Care for Older People: Expectations and recommendations. BGS Compendium, Document C1 (1997).

40. EL(97)3. The Patient's Charter. Privacy and Dignity and the Provision of Single Sex Hospital Accommodation. NHS Executive, 1997.

41. The Royal College of Nursing. Guidelines on Restraint.

42. Bond S. Eating Matters - A Resource for Improving Dietary Care in Hospitals. University of Newcastle Centre for Health Service Research and the Institute for the Elderly, 1997.

43. HAS 2000. Not because they are old. An independent inquiry into the care of older people on acute wards in general hospitals. London: DoH, 1998.

44. Home D. Getting Better? Inspection of Hospital Discharge Arrangements for Older People. SSI/DoH, 1998.

45. Clinical Negligence Scheme for Trusts. CNST Risk Management Standards and Procedures Manual of Guidance, Bristol: CNST, 1996.

46. Health Services Accreditation. Service Standards for Emergency Medical Admissions. Battle: HSA, 1997; Section 8.6.

47. Carers (Recognition and Services) Act. London: HMSO, 1995.

48. George M. Flexible Friends. Community Care 1995; July 20-26.

49. Arksey H et al. Tell it like it is. HSJ 1998; January 22.

50. HSC(98)159: LAC(98)22. Modernising Health and Social Services: National Priorities Guidance. 1999/00-2001/02. September, 1998.

51. Department of Health, Welsh Office. Code of Practice, Mental Health Act 1983.

52. HC(90)22. A Guide to Consent for Examination or Treatment. London: DoH, 1996.

53. Croner. Health Service Risks. 1996.

54. Caldicott Committee. Report on the Review of Patient-Identifiable Information. DoH, 1997.

55. EL(95)37. Activity on Complaints.

56. EL(96)19. Implementation of the new complaints procedure, final guide.

57. Ebrahim S. Ethnic Elders. British Medical Journal 1996; 313.

58. Special Care Group, Department of Health. They look after their own, don't they? Inspection of Community Care Services for Black and Ethnic Minority Older People. DoH/SSI, 1998.

59. Lewisham Hospital NHS Trust. Health Services Research and Evaluation Unit. Lambeth, Southwark and Lewisham Health Commission. Health and Culture Information File. Undated.

60. The Abuse of Older People in Hospital: Information for Workers. Action on Elder Abuse, 1998.

61. East Sussex Multi-Agency Guidelines for the Protection of Vulnerable Adults. 1996.

62. Kingston P, and Phillipson C. Elder Abuse and Neglect. British Journal of Nursing 1994.

63. Craig Y (ed). Elder Abuse and Mediation. Advocacy, Counselling and Mediation in Casework, 1998.

64. Health Services Accreditation. Standards for Care of the Dying. Battle: HSA, 1996.

65. Bates T, et al. The St Thomas's Hospital Terminal Care Support Team. The Lancet 1981.

66. Dyer C. UK Public Calls for Legislation over Living Wills. BMJ 1998; 316.

67. NHS Centre for Reviews and Dissemination and Nuffield Institute for Health. Preventing falls and subsequent injury in older people. Effective Health Care 1996; 2: 1-16.

68. Department of Health/SSI. Assessing Older People with Dementia Living in the Community. London: DoH, 1996.

69. The Royal College of Speech and Language Therapists. Communicating Quality II. London: RCSLT, 1996.

70. Setting New Standards: Bulletin on the Impact of New Therapies for Alzheimer's Disease on Health Service Decision Makers. Macmillan Magazines Limited. Undated.

71. Meyer BS. Telling Patients they have Alzheimer's Disease. BMJ 1997; 314.

72. Hunter R, et al. Alzheimer's Disease in the UK: Developing Patient and Carer Support Strategies to Encourage Care in the Community. Quality in Health Care 1997; 6: 146-152.

73. Clinical Standards Advisory Group. Report on Clinical Effectiveness using Stroke Care as an Example. London: HMSO, 1998.

74. The Royal College of Physicians. Stroke Audit Package - produced by the UK Stroke Audit Group and the Royal College of Physicians. London: 1994.

Appendix IV - Other consulted sources

In and Out of Hospital. Positive Publications.

Carpenter I, Calnan M. Grey Matters. Health Service Journal. January, 1997.

British Geriatric Society. Compendium Document. Sections A-G. BGS. 1997.

National Carers Association - Carers Code.

Henwood M. Ignored and invisible? Carers' experience of the NHS. Carers National Association. June, 1998.

A Better Home Life. CPA. 1996.

Clinical Guidelines by Consensus for Speech and Language Therapists. Royal College of Speech and Language Therapists. May, 1998.

Young J B, Foster A. The Bradford Community Stroke Trial. Results at Six Months. BMJ 1992; 304: 1085-1091.

Oakley A, et al. Preventing Falls and Subsequent Injury in Older People. Quality in Health Care 1996; 5: 243-249.

Good Practice Identified by Research Care Management Practice. Series No.2. Care Plan. March, 1996.

Health and Safety at Work Act. London: HMSO, 1974.

Manual Handling Operations Regulations. London: HMSO, 1992.

Management of Health and Safety at Work Regulations. London: HMSO, 1992.

Chartered Society of Physiotherapy. Standards of Good Practice. The Association of Chartered Physiotherapists in the Community. London: 1995.

Age Concern. Inquiry into Long-Term Care - Evidence to the Health Select Committee. Paper 2. April, 1995.

Wilson A. Being Heard. Report of the Review Committee on NHS Complaints Procedures. HMSO, 1994.

NHS Management Executive. Arrangements Between Health Authorities and NHS Trusts and Private and Voluntary Sector Organisations for the Provision of Community Care Services. HSG (95)45.

Royal College of Nursing. Standards, nutrition and the older adult. London: RCN, 1993.

McWhirter J P, Pennington R. Incidence and recognition of malnutrition in hospital. BMJ 308: 9 April 1994.

Appendix V - Safety and Efficacy Register of New Interventional Procedures (SERNIP)

New interventional procedures in medicine are being developed with considerable speed. These have major implications for patient safety and medical education. The Department of Health is therefore giving its full support to an initiative led by the Academy of Medical Royal Colleges to establish an "intelligence centre" for new interventional procedures.

The Safety and Efficacy Register of New Interventional Procedures (SERNIP) will register new procedures and co-ordinate the experiences of clinicians developing new techniques, allowing data to be rapidly accessed by other clinicians. This is a voluntary system, designed to support innovation and good professional practice in groups undertaking novel procedures. It is important that doctors should be able to show that what they are doing is safe and effective.

SERNIP is initially open to surgical, gynaecological, radiological and cardiological procedures. It supports the Department's philosophy for a research and knowledge-based culture in the NHS. It will work hand-in-hand with the Standing Group on Health Technology to evaluate new procedures where research is felt to be an important requirement in determining whether a new interventional procedure should be introduced into health service practice.

Clinicians planning to pilot procedures which are not listed in the NHS Read Codes should contact SERNIP who will classify procedures as follows:

a. Safety and efficacy established; procedure may be used
b. Sufficiently close to a procedure of established safety and efficacy to give no reasonable grounds for questioning safety and efficacy; procedure may be used
c. Safety and efficacy not yet established; procedure requires a fully-controlled evaluation and may be used only as part of systematic research, comprising either an observational study or a randomised, controlled trial
d. Safety and/or efficacy shown to be unsatisfactory; procedure should not be used.

SERNIP will receive enquiries from those wishing to undertake a procedure and will notify them promptly of its current status. SERNIP will also receive information on new interventional procedures from Royal Colleges and the NHS Central Research and Development Committee's (CRDC) Standing Group on Health Technology (SGHT).

Further information is available from the Administrator, Safety and Efficacy Register of New Interventional Procedures, The Academy of Medical Royal Colleges, 1 Wimpole Street, London W1M 8AE (Tel: 0171 290 3917, Fax: 0171 290 3914).

Annex A - Sample Accreditation Statements

As the basis for its complementary Accreditation Instrument, the HSA report on Service Standards for the NHS Care of Older People is distilled into statements which define and describe its chief characteristics. The following samples are presented as in illustration of method and content.

Statements printed in standard type are 'minimum' standards, which must be applicable to your service if it is to deliver safe and effective care. Statements printed in italic type are 'best practice' and their application to your service will indicate the extent to which it features innovation and excellence.

Each statement is followed by a section reference number which relates it to its source(s) in the report.

CARE SERVICES IN THE COMMUNITY:

THE REFERRAL OF OLDER PEOPLE TO COMMUNITY HEALTH SERVICES

Whether referred by their primary health care team, or by their acute Trust on their discharge from hospital, whether self-referring or referred by their carers or any other service, older people referred to their local community health services have the assurance that their general practitioner will be informed of the fact and given a written report on their assessment; they themselves will be fully informed of the reason(s) for their referral and their consent will have been sought; and their referral correspondence will have contained all essential information. As a result older people can be confident that their referrals will be handled efficiently to facilitate their speedy and appropriate access to care. (2.2.1, 2.2.2, 2.2.3)

SERVICES AVAILABLE TO OLDER PEOPLE IN THE COMMUNITY

Services available in the community include the full range of health and social care services judged to be essential by the service standards report if older people are to be assured access to appropriate and adequate domiciliary care, whether resident at home or in nursing or residential establishments. The identity and accessibility of each of these services is made known to the others and to the public. (2.3.1, 2.3.2)

HOSPITAL BASED SERVICES:

ENSURING THE NUTRITION AND HYDRATION OF OLDER PATIENTS

It is essential that all services providing inpatient care for older people recognise and adequately respond to the risk of inadequate nutrition and dehydration. The service standards set out means of ensuring older patients are assessed for nutritional deficiencies or associated difficulties, e.g. swallowing; that responsibility for the question of nutrition and ensuring patients eat and drink is identified to named staff; that nutritious, attractive and culturally appropriate meals are regularly and conveniently provided, and that guidelines for parenteral nutrition are adopted and observed. This service achieves these standards and ensures its older patients receive adequate nutrition and hydration. (3.10.1 - 3.10.9)

COMMUNICATING BETWEEN SERVICES

COMMUNICATION ON DISCHARGE FROM HOSPITAL

The scope for serious breakdowns in patient care following the discharge of older people from hospital is considerable. Hence the assessment of complex needs and the preparation of multi-disciplinary care plans for meeting older patients' needs in the community must begin as early as possible into the inpatient episode. Overseeing assessment and care planning must be the designated responsibility of identified staff. It is essential that notices giving discharge and patient information to general practitioners and other service providers are promptly dispatched and satisfy minimum data-set requirements. Older people discharged from this inpatient facility are assured that systems are in place which ensure these standards are met. (4.7.1 - 4.7.6)

MAINTAINING THE PATIENT'S DIGNITY

RECOGNISING AND RESPONDING TO THE ABUSE OF OLDER PEOPLE
Those providing health or social services to older people are well placed to identify instances of elder abuse and institute means of remedy and redress. Care services should all work to joint, cross-service policies addressing the detection, investigation, assessment and best response to the abuse of older people, proposing agreed strategies for the recognition of warning signs in domestic, institutional or hospital settings, and offering guidance on appropriate action to counter it where found. Older people cared for by this service are protected by the implementation of such policies. (5.5.1-5.5.10)

STRATEGIES FOR RESPONDING TO THE ISSUE OF FALLS

A STRATEGY FOR PREVENTING FALLS IN THE COMMUNITY SETTING
Unintentional injury, most often caused by a fall, is the sixth leading cause of death among older people. General practitioners, health visitors or other formal care providers encountering older people in the course of their duties must ensure they identify those at risk of falling and sponsor a multi-professional assessment of that risk, adopting a management pathway which addresses all clinical or social risks of falling. It is the policy of service providers in this locality to do this. (6.1.2-6.1.5)

Annex B - Accreditation Instrument for Service Standards for the NHS Care of Older People

Using the Service Standards for the NHS Care of Older People report as the foundation, Health Services Accreditation will develop a companion accreditation instrument which draws upon the principal elements in the report and expresses them as quality defining statements. The applicability of each statement to your service depends upon the achievement of a number of standards, and for each standard the accreditation instrument sets out precisely what evidence is required to show that it is met in practice.

Accreditation instruments have two purposes. First, they act as a vehicle for the explicit and objective external validation of your service's quality. They are designed to avoid confusion by being specific about the type of evidence required. They also serve to eliminate any subjectivity or bias from the accreditation process.

Second, outlining in greater detail the characteristics of a quality service, they also serve as a manual for service improvement. They not only highlight where action may need to be taken but also identify what the action should be.

This annex takes a close look at two sample accreditation statements with their supplementary standards and required evidence, taken from Service Standards for the NHS Care of Older People, showing the approach HSA adopts and the thinking behind the method.

❶ The Statement
Each accreditation item is introduced by a statement focusing on a particular area or aspect of the service under consideration. For a statement to be applied to your service you will be required to achieve one or more subsidiary standards, as in this example. The statement's applicability to your service is given above in the box, in a note which identifies the statement's status in terms of a minimum or best practice standard of service.

❷ Guidance for the reader
To make the accreditation instruments easy to use, guidance is provided on which sections of the service standards report the statement is based.

❸ Subsidiary standards and evidence required
For a statement to be applied to a service, a number of different but related standards first have to be achieved. The subsidiary standards are expressed as sub-sections of the overall standards statement. The type and quantity of evidence required may vary, according to the range or degree of specified policy or activity contained in the report. The evidence required may range from evidence of the policy; the demonstration of the availability of processes, procedures and facilities; the implementation of policy or adoption of procedures and guidelines in practice; into actual measurement of performance or outcome.

❹ Evidence required - policy
The agreement and setting down of policy, aims and objectives is often the first step towards a safe and effective service. It follows that the first items of evidence required are often written policies, demonstrating that issues have been formally and thoughtfully addressed and a clear focus for action identified.

⑤ Evidence required - policy is implemented
When appropriate, the instrument will look for evidence that the service is implementing its policy.

⑥ Evidence required - process and procedure
Once the policy has been determined, the instrument seeks evidence that the procedures, structures or facilities etc., required to enable staff to implement the policy are in place.

⑦ Written evidence in advance
Evidence may be required in written form which will be submitted to HSA in advance of the Accreditation Visit. HSA will evaluate it against the specifications set out in the service standards report.

⑧ Evidence required - measurement of performance or outcome
In some cases the instrument only seeks evidence that systems are in place and underway for the audit/monitoring measurement of the performance of the service.

⑨ Evidence sought on-site by the Accreditation Visitor(s)
The Accreditation Visitor(s) perform three functions when visiting your site. They may (as here) seek confirmation that your service/facilities/organisation etc. are as you describe; they may test the evidence of performance provided by audit by on-site investigation, audit or survey; they may collect new information/evidence, as specifically identified in the accreditation instrument.

⑩ Subsidiary standard - achievement
Only if all the preceding evidence has been confirmed as present can the subsidiary standard be shown as achieved. This is recorded as shown here.

Statements achieved - accreditation report
For a statement to be confirmed as applying to your service, and thus credited to your accreditation report, each of its supporting subsidiary standards must be achieved. The statements which are applicable are then recorded and published in a report prepared at the end of the accreditation process and placed in the public domain.

Statement: Strategies for responding to the issue of falls

A strategy for preventing falls in the community setting

It is essential that this statement, representing a 'minimum' standard of service, applies to your service:

Unintentional injury, most often caused by a fall, is the sixth leading cause of death among older people. General practitioners, health visitors or other formal care providers encountering older people in the course of their duties must ensure they identify those at risk of falling and sponsor a multi-professional assessment of that risk, adopting a management pathway which addresses all clinical or social risks of falling. It is the policy of service providers in this locality to do this.

(6.1.2-6.1.5)

This statement is based on section 6.1 of the report.

This statement will be credited to your accreditation report provided the evidence is forthcoming to confirm that the following two standards are met in practice. You may use the (✔) box against each item of evidence to record your progress as you prepare evidence or submit it to HSA or, in the case of evidence which is to be verified by the Accreditation Visitor(s), your certainty that this evidence is actually available on site.

1.
Standard

NHS staff conducting health checks or home visits on persons over 75 years of age are aware of the importance of screening their patients for indicators of falls risk, and organise a comprehensive assessment of their risk of falls for these patients.

1.1   The Community Care Trust undertaking this accreditation is required to demonstrate that it has prompted or participated in the drawing up of a falls prevention strategy for its catchment area. It will therefore be expected to produce a written falls prevention policy, with evidence that this was developed in collaboration with the primary health care team, the local acute hospital's department of geriatric medicine and accident and emergency department, and social services.

(✔)
☐

1.2   The Community Care Trust must produce evidence to HSA which demonstrates that this policy has been shared among all the services represented in the drafting of the policy, e.g. all local primary health care teams, social services, acute Trusts (especially accident and emergency departments, departments of geriatric medicine, directorates of surgery).

(✔)
☐

1.3   The written policy must identify the principal indicators of risk of falling set out in section 6.1.3 of the standards report, and go on to outline the procedures by which persons identified by screening as being at risk of falling are then offered and given a falls risk assessment which includes a review of their living environment.

(✔)
☐

1.4   Evidence that older patients are screened for indicators of "risk of falling" when they come into contact with health care and social services staff, and are then appropriately fully assessed (when this is indicated) will consist of a copy of the screening and assessment documentation in use for this purpose locally by the health and social care providers listed under item 1.2 above. The documentation will be expected to include reference to the indicators detailed in section 6.1.3 and the assessments listed in sections 6.1.4 and 6.1.5 of the report.

(✔)
☐

For HSA use:	YES	NO
This Service meets Standard 1	☐	☐

2.

> **Standard**
>
> **The local strategy for prevention of falls among older people seeks to ensure that each patient benefits from an individually tailored falls prevention assessment (if the need is established).**

2.1   The policy referred to under item 1.1 above stipulates that all persons identified as at risk of falling on their being screened for the presence of risk indicators, or who have come into contact with the NHS as a result of an unexplained fall or repeated falls, must receive a full, medical assessment designed to identify all treatable causes of their fall(s), conducted by their general practitioner.

(✔)
☐

2.2   The policy goes on to require that if the patient is being assessed as a result of having had a fall, and no treatable medical reason for the fall is identified, the patient should still benefit from an occupational therapy/physiotherapy assessment, including a home visit, where that is appropriate.

(✔)
☐

	YES	NO
For HSA use: **This Service meets Standard 2**	☐	☐

Statement: Hospital based services

Ensuring the nutrition and hydration of older patients

It is essential that this statement, representing a 'minimum' standard of service, applies to your service:

It is essential that all services providing inpatient care for older people recognise and adequately respond to the risk of inadequate nutrition and dehydration. The service standards set out means of ensuring older patients are assessed for nutritional deficiencies or associated difficulties e.g. swallowing; that responsibility for the question of nutrition and ensuring patients eat and drink is identified to named staff; that nutritious, attractive and culturally appropriate meals are regularly and conveniently provided, and that guidelines for parenteral nutrition are adopted and observed. This service achieves these standards and ensures its older patients receive adequate nutrition and hydration.

(3.10.1 - 3.10.9)

This statement is based on section 3.10 of the report.

This statement will be credited to your accreditation report provided the evidence is forthcoming to confirm that the following four standards are met in practice. You may use the (✔) box against each item of evidence to record your progress as you prepare evidence or submit it to HSA or, in the case of evidence which is to be verified by the Accreditation Visitor(s), your certainty that this evidence is actually available on site.

1.

Standard

Older patients are assessed for their nutritional status on admission to hospital.

1.1   The Trust must supply HSA with a copy of a set of guidelines/protocol applied to all cases of admission of older people, designed to identify any inadequate nutritional status, assess their nutritional risk and screen them for swallowing problems.

(✔)
☐

1.2   These guidelines/protocol must carry the written endorsement of the Trust dietetics service and must inform the user that the dietetics service is available for advice on individual patients within 24 hours of a patient being referred to them.

(✔)
☐

1.3   The hospital must confirm to HSA in a written statement from the Director of Nursing that it is Trust policy to ensure that at least one nurse on each ward receiving older people has a special interest in nutrition.

(✔)
☐

1.4   The guidelines/protocol (which must carry the written endorsement of the speech and language therapy department) must contain prompts for screening for swallowing problems and set out the procedure for referring patients identified as having these problems to the speech and language therapist. The guidelines/protocol must confirm that the speech and language therapist will assess patients referred to them within no longer than two working days from receipt of the referral.

(✔)
☐

	YES	NO
For HSA use: **This Service meets Standard 1**	☐	☐

2.

> ### Standard
>
> **Older people are provided with nutritious, attractive, regularly served and culturally appropriate meals.**

2.1   The Trust's hotel services/catering department is requested to provide HSA with a copy of its catering policy (or some other written and publicly available material) in which it explicitly states its intention of meeting this standard and sets out what it does in order to do so (e.g. vegetarian or other alternative menus, flexible meal times, snack meals or nutritious drinks available on the wards at any time etc.).   (✔) ☐

2.2   HSA must be sent the timetable for meals served on wards. This will be expected to show that the interval between the last main meal (not snack) of the day and breakfast never exceeds fourteen (14) hours.   (✔) ☐

	YES	NO
For HSA use: **This Service meets Standard 2**	☐	☐

3.

> **Standard**
>
> **Procedures for the delivery of parenteral nutrition are never denied to older patients on the grounds of their age.**

3.1   HSA require to see a copy of the protocol in use for the provision of parenteral nutrition to older people. The protocol must carry a statement to the effect that patients must never be denied access to this management on grounds of age.

(✔)
☐

3.2   HSA must also receive a copy of the protocol in use covering the insertion of gastronomy (PEG) tubes and the management of percutaneous endoscopic gastronomy. Again this protocol must also carry a statement to the effect that access to this procedure must be based on clinical need and never denied on grounds of age.

(✔)
☐

3.3   The management of percutaneous endoscopic gastronomy according to this protocol (3.2) should be subject to routine clinical audit. HSA should be sent a copy of an audit report on the management of percutaneous endoscopic gastronomy arising from an audit conducted within the twelve months preceding the accreditation visit.

8

(✔)
☐

	YES	NO
For HSA use: **This Service meets Standard 3**	☐	☐

<table>
<tr><td>

4.

</td><td>

Standard

It is applied policy of the department of geriatric medicine that particular care is taken to ensure that all their patients are appropriately and adequately fed.

</td></tr>
</table>

4.1   HSA must be sent a copy of the department of geriatric medicine's written policy on general nutrition and nutritional support. This policy will be required to contain explicit reference to the crucial importance of ensuring all their patients receive appropriate and adequate nutrition and hydration.

(✔)
☐

4.2   The policy must highlight the special attention which must be given to assisting acutely confused patients to eat and drink.

(✔)
☐

4.3   The policy must include reference to measures for ensuring all patients are given the aid they need to feed themselves at meal times.

(✔)
☐

4.4   The policy will require the induction or continuing education of nursing and medical staff appointed to the department of geriatric medicine to include reference to general nutrition, the techniques of nutritional support and the department's policy on ensuring all patients are fed.

(✔)
☐

4.5   The policy will stipulate that it is the responsibility of each patient's named nurse to ensure that arrangements are in place which guarantee the patient's nutrition and ability to eat or drink are taken care of.

(✔)
☐

4.6   The Accreditation Visitors will audit patient's notes seeking confirmation that they contain records of the patient's nutritional status assessment, notes on their ability to eat and drink, any special arrangements to assist them in this respect and a record of their eating and drinking (meals completed, dietary supplements taken etc.).

(✔)
☐

9

10

	YES	NO
For HSA use: **This Service meets Standard 4**	☐	☐

Notes